Integrated Diseases Management

NIPA® GENX ELECTRONIC RESOURCES & SOLUTIONS P. LTD.
New Delhi-110 034

Integrated Disease Management Principles and Practices

Sanjeev Kumar
Assistant Professor/Scientist
Department of Plant Pathology
Office of Dean, Faculty of Agriculture
Jawaharlal Nehru Krishi Vishwa Vidyalaya
Jabalpur-482004, Madhya Pradesh, India

NIPA® GENX ELECTRONIC RESOURCES & SOLUTIONS P. LTD.
New Delhi-110 034

NIPA® GENX ELECTRONIC
RESOURCES & SOLUTIONS P. LTD.
101,103, Vikas Surya Plaza, CU Block
L.S.C.Market, Pitam Pura, New Delhi-110 034
Ph : +91 11 27341616, 27341717, 27341718
E-mail:newindiapublishingagency@gmail.com
Website: www.nipabooks.com

For customer assistance, please contact
Phone: + 91-11-27 34 17 17
Fax: + 91-11-27 34 16 16
E-Mail: feedbacks@nipabooks.com

ISBN: 978-93-95319-18-8

Composed and Designed by NIPA®.

About The Author

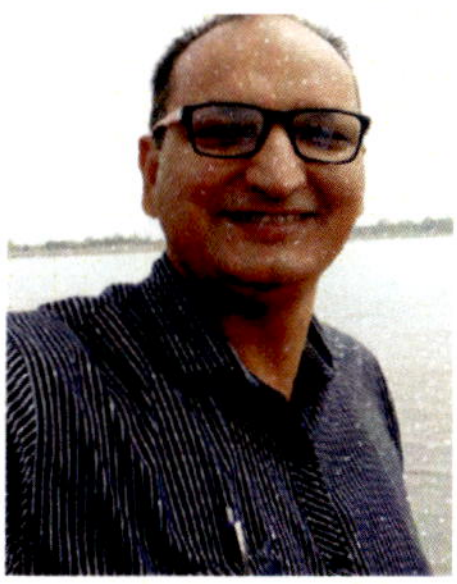

Dr. Sanjeev Kumar is Assistant Professor/Scientist, Department of Plant Pathology, Jawaharlal Nehru Krishi Vishwavidyalaya, Jabalpur, Madhya Pradesh. He is very sincere and hard working teacher. He has taught many undergraduate, postgraduate and Ph.D courses with great dedication to the great satisfaction of the students and actively involved in all teaching activities. Dr. Kumar has guided 20 M.Sc and 1 Ph.D student and has been actively involved in his research and extension activities too. As a researcher, he has been associated with 8 major research projects sponsored by ICAR, NATP,TSP and JICA, Japan. He has published 68 research and reviews papers, 25 book chapters, 105 popular articles, 1 research bulletin and 3 technical folders. He is an active member of over six National and International Societies. He is the fellow member of Indian Phytopathological Society, IARI New Delhi, Indian Society of Mycology and Plant Pathology, Udaipur, Rajasthan and Society of Biocontrol Advancement, Banguluru. He has attended many conferences, symposia, workshops and presented papers. He has also attended the World Soybean Research Conference held in Durban, South Africa.

Dr. Kumar has authored seven books entitled Plant Pathogens & Principles of Plant Pathology, Diseases of Horticultural Crops: Identification & Management, Diseases of Field Crops and their Integrated Management, Pesticides and Plant Protection Appliances and Diseases of Field & Horticultural Crops & Their Management-II Fundamentals of Plant Pathology published by New India Publishing Agency, New Delhi and Textbook of Diseases of Field & Horticultural Crops & Their Management-I, published by Brillion Publishing, New Delhi – 110005 and three practical manuals. His research interests include pulse pathology and biological control.

Preface

The Indian Council of Agricultural Research (ICAR), New Delhi an apex body developed new course curricula for Undergraduate and Post graduate students under the umbrella of 6th Dean's & BSMA Committee. The syllabus has been completely revised and has rendered existing textbooks obsolete or incomplete for students. This gap in knowledge give me an excellent opportunity to present updated textbooks to students as per their syllabus requirements. This book of Integrated Disease Management is a carefully written for UG & PG class and is completely in accordance with the latest syllabus. The purpose of writing this text books is to provide the basic and emerging facts where by the students may be introduced to the scientific foundation of this course Integrated Disease Management. I have taken utmost care to present facts according to the level of our students and graded our content accordingly.

This book has some features of its own, These are:

Fun Time: Sets the tone by addressing general terminology which also relate to the subject. Fun time is good ice breaker and prepares the students for the information to follow.

Info hive: Stimulates the young minds as they look to learn, yet newer things and broaden their horizons.

Text: The text in the book is clear, well presented, sequentially arranged. The chapters are designed in a way that leads to the comprehensive learning of the key concepts, help in the development of the investigative skill of the students.

I wish to express my sincere gratitude to our past and present pioneers in the field of Plant Pathology whose work has been freely used in the creation of this book.

This book is dedicated to my parents, who sacrificed everything to give me the most and best education possible, to my wife, 'Archana' whose love and support have been the most precious things to me throughout our life together, and who helped me in many facets of preparation of this and of previous books and finally, to "Saumya" and "Adyan", our youngest children, who, someday, when they read their names in the book, may be reassured of "Papa" love for them, and may feel proud of their father.

Omission and mistakes are bound to be found in this endeavor and I am prepared to bear the accountability of making any misrepresentation of facts. Teachers and students are requested to comment and give suggestions for further improvements in the book.

Sanjeev Kumar
Jabalpur

February, 2023

Contents

Funtime (Glossary)

Sl No	Name of term	Definition
1.	Action threshold/ Economic threshold	The disease level at which a control tactic must be implemented to avoid an economic loss.
2.	Active Ingredient	The component of a pesticide formulation that affects or kills the target pest or performs the pesticide's function.
3.	Allelopathy	The ability of a plant species to produce substances that are toxic to certain other plants.
4.	Antagonist	An organism that releases toxins or otherwise changes conditions in a way that reduces the activity or growth of other organisms
5.	Augmentative biological control	Release of large numbers of a biological control agent to supplement the small numbers already present, in expectation of a greatly increased effect.
6.	Band application	An application in which pesticide is applied in strips, usually to the planting bed or seed row.
7.	Biodegradation	The breaking down of a substance (e.g., a pesticide) by organisms (commonly microorganisms) in the environment.
8.	Biological control	The use of living organisms, such as predators, parasitoids, and pathogens, to control pest insects, weeds, or diseases.
9.	Biorational	Having a minimal disruptive influence upon the environment and its inhabitants (e.g., a biorational insecticide).
10.	Broadcast application	The application of a substance (e.g. pesticide) to an entire area (e.g., field or orchard).
11.	Classical biological control	The importation of foreign natural enemies to control previously introduced, or native, pests.
12.	Conservation biological control	Any biological control practice designed to protect and maintain populations of existing natural enemies.
13.	Crop protection	Crop protection is the collection of tools, products, and best practices farmers use to protect their crops from the negative impact of weeds, pests and disease.
14.	Crop rotation	The practice of purposefully alternating crop species grown on the same plot of land, typically to improve soil conditions or manage diseases.
15.	Cross resistance	A condition in which a pest population that has developed *resistance* to one type or group of pesticides is also resistant to another type or group of pesticides, even in the absence of exposure to the latter pesticides.

16.	Dossiers	Compilation of all study reports and accompanying documents necessary to register an active substance or a plant protection product.
17.	Economic threshold	The point at which a pest has become numerous or damaging enough to require a management action (e.g., pesticide application) to prevent intolerable economic loss. The point at which the damage caused by a pest exceeds the cost of taking a management action to reduce the pest's abundance or subsequent damage. May also be called *action threshold* or *treatment threshold*.
18.	Environmental impact quotient (EIQ)	A relative value that estimates the environmental impact of a pesticide, by taking into account toxicity to natural enemies, wildlife, and humans, degree of exposure, aquatic and terrestrial effects, soil chemistry, etc.
19.	Exclusion	The act of keeping pests away from crops, structures, or other areas, commonly by using barriers such as fencing, row covers, or screens.
20.	Habitat manipulation	Manipulation of agricultural areas and surrounding environment with the aim of conserving or augmenting populations of natural enemies (e.g., the planting of a refuge for natural enemies).
21.	Hyperparasite	A parasite whose host is another parasite.
22.	Integrated disease management (IDM)	An approach to the management of disease in which all available control options, including physical, chemical, and biological controls, are evaluated and integrated into a unified program.
23.	Inundative release	The release of relatively large numbers of natural enemies to suppress pest populations, without the expectation that the natural enemies will colonize and spread throughout the area.
24.	Microbials	In agriculture, microbial products are those made from microorganisms to help protect crops from disease and pests, and to encourage healthy growth.
25.	Microbial pesticides	A preparation of microorganisms (e.g., viruses or bacteria) or their products used to suppress pest populations.
26.	Monitoring	Carefully gathering and recording information on the abundance, development, and growth of organisms (typically pests or crops) or other factors (e.g., crop damage), often utilizing very specific procedures and commonly on a regular basis over a period of time.
27.	Maximum Residue Level (MRL)	(Maximum Residue Level) The potential residues on a harvested crop are regulated by maximum level.
28.	Natural control	The suppression of pest populations by naturally occurring biological and environmental agents.
29.	Natural enemies	Living organisms found in nature that kill, weaken, or reduce the reproductive potential of other organisms.
30.	Pest resurgence	The rapid rebound of pest abundance after the numbers were reduced by management action.

31.	Pesticide rotation	The practice of alternating pesticides of different modes of action in order to prevent the development of pesticide resistance.
31.	Quarantine	A period of enforced isolation and restricted movement that is imposed to prevent the spread of pests. The legal enforcement of measures aimed to prevent a pest from spreading or establishing in new areas.
32.	Sampling/Scouting	Estimating the density of organisms (pests or natural enemies) or damage by examining a defined portion of the crop.
33.	Sanitation	Activity that reduces the spread of pathogen inoculum, especially the removal and destruction of infected plant parts and cleaning of equipment and tools. The practice of removing crop debris and weeds from growing areas.
34.	Soil Solarization	The practice of heating soil to levels lethal to pests using solar energy by laying clear plastic on soil surfaces for 4 to 6 weeks during warm, sunny weather.
35.	Target disease	The disease that a management action (e.g., a pesticide application) is intended to destroy or manage.
36.	Trap crop	A crop or portion of a crop intended to attract pests so they can be destroyed by treating a relatively small area or by destroying the trap crop and the pests together.
37.	Treatment threshold	The point at which a given disease level is enough that a management action (e.g., a pesticide application) is necessary to prevent economic loss or unacceptable damage. May also be called*action threshold* and *economic threshold*.

Infohive
Current Facts About Crop Protection

1. India is abundant in natural wealth (*AatmNirbhar India*)

- While only 11% of the entire land globally is arable, 56% of our land is arable.
- Sixty four types of soils are available all over the world and India has 46 types of soils.
- We are rich in availability of rain, surface and ground water. We are able to use only 10-15% of our abundant rainfall.
- Of the total land area of 328.7 million hectares, about 30 crore hectares is catchment area. There are about 445 rivers in the country, whose length is about two lakh kilometers.
- Due to excessive water exploitation caused by Green Revolution, today about 264 districts in the country are categorized as dark zone, and are facing water crisis.
- Ground water level is decreasing at the rate of 0.3 meters every year.
- There are 15 types of climate zones globally, and 127 agro-climatic zones, all of which are available in all of India.
- In terms of biodiversity, India has 48,000 varieties of trees, 1500 edible plants and 811 species of domestic and wild animals.
- India has about 375 varieties of fruits, 280 varieties of vegetables, about 80 types of kandamul, about 60 types of flowers, seeds and nuts.
- India has 77 km long coastline and our own economic area of 20 lakh sq km, which offers not only a lot of fishing but also valuable oil, gas, minerals and power generation potential.

2. India : Unique challenges

- Indian agriculture is characterized by small land holdings, highly diverse, heterogeneous , fragmented and not uniform across the states and districts.
- Every 100 kms in any direction, there is change in soil, climate, cropping pattern, languages, food and culture.

- With approximately 110 million farm families spread across 600,000 villages, reaching out and connecting has understandably remained a challenge.
- Indian agriculture lacks cost and quality competitiveness.
- It is not remunerative enough, as 52 % of the total labour force employed in agriculture contributes only 17 % of the GDP.
- India ranks eighth in global exports of agricultural produce with only $ 39 billion of annual exports.
- More and more people are moving out of agriculture.
- The younger generations are not interested to continue unless new innovative products and technologies are offered to make
- Biggest challenge agriculture faces today is the adverse impact of climate change and weather aberrations (abiotic stresses), deteriorating soil health, environmental sustainability.

3. Global & national yield losses due to pests, pathogens and weeds

- Pests, pathogens, and weeds are responsible for 20–40% loss of global agricultural productivity.
- In India, 20-25% crop losses are reported due to pest attacks every year.
- As per Ministry of Agriculture, India is losing agricultural production worth INR 1.48 lakh crores annually due to damage from pests, weeds and plant diseases.

4. Crop protection is in constant evolution

- Climate change is an important development that has affected global population and agriculture.
- Complexity of pests is, likely to increase, with more frequent pest outbreaks.
- Pest and disease dynamics have altered considerably.
- Many minor pests have become major pests and many new pest and diseases have emerged.
- This has kept the crop protection sector on their toes.
- There are strengths and opportunities for updating existing approaches of pest management.
- Public and private sectors will be keen on investing in better delivery techniques and products that leave very little impact on the plant and the soil.

5. Pesticides: Play vital role in raising food production

- Almost 20-40% of the world's potential crop production is lost annually due to effect of weeds, pests and diseases.

- Crop losses would be doubled if the existing pesticide use would be abandoned, significantly sending food prices to roof.
- Even after the harvest, crops are at the risk of being damaged.
- Pesticides have changed drastically over the year to become much safer for both human and environment.
- Use of pesticide in India is only 460 grams per hectare whereas in China it is 6 Kg per hectare.
- Agriculture land in India is 148 million hectares whereas in China the farm land is 128 million hectares. However, China is using 4-5 times more pesticides than India .
- India's total food production is valued at $400 Bn whereas China's food production is over $1000 Bn.
- This only proves that pesticides play an important role in raising the food production in a country.

6. Status of Pesticides in India

- Only 294 products are registered in India.
- Pakistan, Vietnam etc have more than 500 pesticides.
- USA has more than 850 products and China has more than 1000 products registered.
- About 50% of the molecules used in India are more than 20-40 years old.
- It take 5-8 years for a new molecule to be registered.
- There is no original research or innovation done on pesticides molecules in our country.
- More than 95% of pesticide molecules' technology is imported. It is introduced in the country by local manufacturers.
- The process of registration and generating data of a new molecule takes 5-7 years.
- It calls for investment of Rs 30-40 crore. In addition, the company has to spend Rs 50-100 crore for product launch, education and training of farmers and commercialization of the product.

7. India : Among the lowest user of pesticide in the world.

- Domestic market has enormous growth potential because of low pesticide use, which is among the lowest in the world.
- India's per hectare consumption of pesticide stands at 0.6kg/ha against the global average consumption of 3kg/ha.
- Increase in pesticide consumption and bringing hitherto untapped areas of cultivation under its umbrella will help to boost agriculture productivity and feed our increasing population and *doubling farmers' income* by 2022.

8. Need to increased usage of crop protection products

- India is the most dynamic and largest generic manufacturer of agrochemicals in the world.
- It has about 75 technical grade pesticides manufacturers and more than 600 formulators.
- This enables farmers, mainly poor farmers, to get crop protection products at a very low price.
- At present, only 25-30% cultivated area is covered by the crop protection umbrella. There is need for increased usage of crop protection products.

9. Changing dynamics of pesticides in India

- India is the fourth-largest producer of crop protection products globally after the United States, Japan, and China.
- Domestic market was estimated at Rs 23,200 Cr for 2020. It is projected to reach a value of Rs 31,600 Cr by 2024, growing at CAGR of 8.1 % during 2019-2024.
- Domestic market, insecticides have a 44 per cent share. Fungicides and herbicides almost have an equal share of around 22% each. The balance 12% is represented by plant growth regulators, bio-stimulants, seed treatment segments.
- Total pesticide consumption is the highest in Maharashtra, followed by Uttar Pradesh, Punjab, and Haryana.
- While insecticides dominate the Indian crop protection market forming the highest share, fungicide and herbicides are emerging as the fastest-growing segment.

10. Impact of pesticides in Agriculture

- Globally, about 1/3 of agricultural products depend on pesticides.
- Without the use of pesticides, there could be a
  - 78% loss in fruit production.
  - 54% loss in vegetable production.
  - 32% loss in cereal production.

11. Share of pesticides in cost of cultivation

- Commenting on the affordability of CPP, Dr Dalwai Committee report, on "Doubling Farmers Income" mentions that cost of pesticides is only 0.4% of total cost incurred by the farmers.
- The share of pesticides in the cost of cultivation was
  - 3 per cent in cotton.

- 1.9 per cent in paddy.
- Further lower in wheat (0.7%) and sugarcane (0.3%).

12. Ban on 27 pesticides

- Ban pesticides are: Acephate, Atrazine, Benfuracarb, Butachlor, Captan, Carbendazim, Carbofuran, Chlorpyriphos, 2,4-D, Deltamethrin, Dicofol, Dimethoate, Dinocap, Diuron, Malathion, Mancozeb, Methomyl, Monocrotophos, Oxyfluorfen, Pendimethalin, Quinalphos, Sulfosulfuron, Thiodicarb, Thiophanate methyl, Thiram, Zineb, Ziram.
- The 27 generic pesticides proposed to be banned account for 40 per cent of the domestic market and 50 per cent of all exports from India.
- Almost all these pesticides are being used in sizable quantities in most countries including USA, Brazil, China, Australia, New Zealand etc. Many are also used in Europe. Why does India want to ban them?
- India exports almost these pesticides worth Rs 4500 crores to various countries. China will grab this business if we ban these pesticides.
- These are very economical, efficacious and safe products being used for 20-25 years or more.

13. Spurious products are harming crops

- Presence of spurious pesticides in the market result in losses of yield and farmers' income.
- 30% of plant protection chemicals sold in India are spurious.
- There are more than 6,000 agro-chemical companies in India.
- Most of them are not running as per the guidelines of CIB&RC which allows prosecution – but it isn't happening.
- Use of spurious pesticides is growing at about 20% every year.
- Uttar Pradesh, Madhya Pradesh, Maharashtra, Andhra Pradesh, Karnataka, Haryana and West Bengal are among the worst-affected States.
- As per research done by Indian Institute of Public Administration with the help of Ministry of Consumer Affairs, 58% of agri inputs are fake in rural India.
- There are over 1,400 pesticide manufacturing units in India.
- Juxtaposed with poor enforcement of Insecticide Act and Insecticides Rules (1971), this has led to proliferation of spurious and sub-standard products and helps flyby- night operators .

14. Problems due to Spurious/Substandard pesticides

- Crops suffer yield losses due to ineffectiveness of these products in controlling pests.

- Financial loss, indebtedness, distress to farmers.
- Inadequate plant protection impacts national food security.
- Generate unwanted residue on fruits, vegetables and other food commodities.
- Corner major market share of pesticide industry.
- Major revenue loss to GOI in the form of GST and other taxes.
- Contaminate the fields and environment.

15. Farmer awareness

- Farmers must be made aware of the types of illegal pesticides.
- These include:
- Counterfeit pesticides packaged and labelled to look like legal products.
- Counterfeit pesticides with poor or limited labelling and packaging, clearly different from the original.
- Pesticide products without registration in India.
- Nearly 700 KVKs and extension systems working in PPP mode are required to consistently spread awareness regarding the risks posed by use of illegal pesticides.
- PMB 2020 must provide for spreading literacy about buying the right product with bill.

16. Changing dynamics of bio pesticides in India

- Green chemical agents.
- Biopesticides have the potential to work as an alternative to chemical pesticides or along with them, which is essential for sustainable agriculture.
- It is high time to increase the application of biopesticides in the agriculture in order to achieve increasing food demand along with assured food safety.
- Global demand for biopesticides is increasing daily due to consumer awareness regarding food safety.
- Worldwide biopesticides market is projected to grow at a CAGR of 14.7% from an estimated value of USD 4.3 billion in 2020 to reach USD 8.5 billion by 2025.
- As per the reports of market research firm markets and markets, Indian biopesticide market is expected to deliver $778 million by 2025 at a CAGR of 25.4%.
- As per the report of another market research firm Mordor intelligence Market share of biopesticides in India is about 4.5% of total pesticides sale.
- Fruit and vegetable segment are started shifting towards the biopesticides due to increasing food safety concerns from consumer end.

17. Green technology pesticides; Must reach all farmers

- Role of crop protection solutions insures a farmer's investment on other inputs.
- It also ensures the food, nutrition, health, wealth and environment security of the nation.
- We need to strengthen our farmers by providing them latest technology i.e.
  - Green technology pesticides.
  - Only used a few grams per hectare.
  - Much safer for humans, animals and the environment.
  - Minimize the burden of chemicals in agriculture and environment.
  - Spraying through drones.
  - Government's vision: Ensuring the reach of latest technology to even the most marginal farmers.

18. How ICT works in plant pathology

- In case of crop disease, farmer clicks a picture of the diseased foliage.
- Uploads image on the central repository.
- Scientists and plant pathologists study data and analyze it.
- Crop disease is identified by experts.
- Feedback and remedies are shared with farmer via phone.

19. Benefits of ICT

- Easy access to expert opinions.
- Instant identification of plant disease before it spreads.
- Crop loss minimization.
- Profit maximization.
- Easy scalability.
- Simple to use.

20. Digital technologies: Dramatically changing face of plant protection

- Digital penetration in the agri sector is growing at a fast pace!
- Internet
- Mobile technologies
- Drone
- Data analytics
- Artificial Intelligence (AI)
- Big Data

- Block Chain
- Geographical Information Systems (GIS)
- Agriculture Internet of Things (AIoT)
- Apps
- With internet and mobile penetration at the level of 50% and 79% respectively, providing digitally enabled One Stop Solution to the farmers.

1

Plant Health

Plant health

The term "plant health" has two overlapping meanings. In the more specific meaning, plant health refers to plant quarantine, while in the less specific use, it covers all areas of plant protection, such as plant pest management, plant quarantine, and pesticide regulation and application.

Contribution of plant health to food security

There are four ways in which plant health contributes to food security.

1. Contribution to food availability
2. Contribution to food accessibility.
3. Contribution to food affordability.
4. Contribution to food safety.

1. Contribution to food availability

- Food crops are attacked by over 1,000 species of plant pests.
- Crop losses are estimated to make up 10–16 percent of global harvest annually as a result of plant pests damage.
- Meanwhile, crop yields can be recovered by 10-30 percent or even 50 percent through effective implementation of plant health measures.

2. Contribution to food accessibility

- Plant health, and in particular, plant quarantine, directly contributes to promoting food accessibility though trade facilitation.
- Thirty seven international standards for phytosanitary measures (ISPMs), have adopted covering areas of principles, export and imports, surveillance, risk analysis, diagnostics, and treatments.
- Through the implementation of all these standards, global food trade has been greatly facilitated.

3. Contribution to food affordability

- Plant health promotes food affordability through effective reduction of farmers' economic losses resulted from the damage of plant pests.
- For example, the net economic benefit for farmers is increased by 20-40 percent through effective implementation of integrated crop pest management.
- Plant health also promotes food affordability through effective increase in farmers' income by enhancing the agricultural trade.

4. Contribution to food safety

- Over 70 percent of pesticides are applied to field crops and horticultural plants, which bring about potential risks for food safety.
- Plant health measures could greatly promote food safety through effective implementation of crop Integrated Pest Management (IPM).
- For example, 30-60 percent of pesticide application can be reduced through the application of IPM, which would consequently increase food safety.

Why is plant health important?

- Plants are the source of the air we breathe.
- Plants are the source over 80 % of the food we consume.
- Ensure sustainable agriculture and food systems.
- Protect the environment and ecosystems.
- Healthy plants mean healthier people.
- Therefore, keeping plants healthy is not only important – it is absolutely vital.

Healthy plants are no easy feat

- FAO estimates that up to 40 percent of food crops are lost to plant pests and diseases annually.
- This leaves millions of people without enough food to eat and seriously damages agriculture – the primary source of income for poor rural communities.
- Climate change and human activities have altered ecosystems, reducing biodiversity and creating new niches where pests can thrive.
- International travel and trade, which have tripled in volume in the last decade, can quickly spread pests and diseases around the world causing great damage to native plants and the environment.
- Adding to these challenges, people have turned to pesticides to secure yields in plant production.
- In doing so, there are mounting concerns over the effects of plant protection products on the environment, non-target organisms and human health.

Understanding these challenges, the European Parliament and the Council adopted Regulation (EU) 2016/2031 on protective measures against plant pests in October

2016. The new rules entered into force on 13 December of the same year, and aim to modernise the plant health regime, enhance more effective measures for the protection of the Union's territory and its plants, ensure safe trade, and mitigate the impacts of climate change on the health of crops and forests. The United Nations has also declared 2020 as the "International Year of Plant Health" with the aim of raising global awareness on the importance of protecting plant heath.

What are we doing about it?

Role of public sector

1. Promote public awareness campaigns on the importance of plant health and what everyone can do to protect plants.
2. Invest in plant protection organizations and ensure that they have adequate human and financial resources.
3. Invest more in research related to plant health and in innovative practices and technologies, and provide incentives for the private sector and farmers to do so too.
4. Strengthen monitoring and early warning systems to protect plants and plant health.
5. Align policies and actions with Sustainable Development Goals related to plant health, in particular those aimed at eliminating hunger and malnutrition and reducing poverty and threats to the environment.
6. Ensure that phytosanitary import requirements are based on IPPC standards and are technically justified.
7. Enforce plant health standards and strengthen plant protection capacity.

Role of private sector

- Promote environmentally friendly products and practices for preventing and managing disease & pests.
- Make trading and transportation of plants and plant products safer by complying with international plant health standards and legislation.
- Inform clients that transporting plants and plant products may spread plants pests and diseases – sometimes with devastating results.
- Sustain plant health innovative practices and the use of new technologies to facilitate market access in line with international standards.

Role of farmers/common people and agribusinesses

If you are a farmer or work in an agribusiness, you can have a direct influence on plants, and help to keep them healthy.

- Regularly monitor and report the occurrence of disease & pests on your farms.
- Prevent the spread of pests by using only certified disease free seeds and seedlings.
- Adopt environmentally friendly Integrated pest management programme.
- Take advantage of modern digital technology, such as mobile apps and software to access information about how to prevent and manage plant pests or diseases or report outbreaks.
- Be cautious when taking plants and plant products with you when you travel as they may spread plant pest and diseases.
- Be careful when ordering plants and plant products online or through postal services as small packages can easily bypass regular phytosanitary controls.
- Take daily actions to reduce your environmental impact and actively engage in initiatives to protect and manage natural resources.
- Contribute to the global awareness campaign on #Plant Health

2

Definition, Importance & Categories of Plant Diseases

Disease (literally *dis-ease*) implies *lack of 'comfort 'Deviation from normal functioning.'*

Definition

Disease is *any morphological or physiological abnormality in a plant or any of its parts caused by continuous irritation and results in economic losses to human beings.*

or

Disease in plants defined *as the series of invisible and visible responses of plant cells and tissues to a pathogenic organism or environmental factor that result in adverse changes in the form, function, or integrity of the plant and may lead to partial impairment or death of plant parts or of the entire plant.*

All these definitions indicate that disease

1. Is not a pathogen but it is *caused by a pathogen.*
2. It is not symptom but *results in symptoms.*
3. It is not a condition as the condition results from disease and is not synonymous with it.
4. It is *not an injury.*
5. Cannot be infectious, it is *actually the pathogen* which is *infectious.*
6. Results from *continuous* irritation.
7. Malfunctioning process and this result in some suffering and therefore disease is a *pathological process.*

Concept of disease in plants

I. Healthy plant

- A plant is healthy, or normal, when it can carry out its physiological functions to the best of its genetic potential.

- Meristematic (cambium) cells of a healthy plant divide and differentiate as needed.
- Different types of specialized cells absorb water and nutrients from the soil, translocate these to all plant parts.
- Carry on photosynthesis, translocate, metabolize, or store the photosynthetic products.
- Produce seed or other reproductive organs for survival and multiplication.

II. Diseased plant

It is difficult to pinpoint exactly when a plant is diseased because

- It is not known whether plants feel pain or discomfort.
- Plants do not speak,or otherwise communicate with us.
- When the ability of the cells of a plant or plant part to carry out one or more of essential functions is interfered with by either a pathogenic organism or an adverse environmental factor, the activities of the cells are disrupted, altered, or inhibited, the cells malfunction or die, and the plant becomes diseased.
- At first, the affliction is localized to one or a few cells and is invisible.
- Soon, the reaction becomes more widespread and affected plant parts develop changes visible to the naked eye.

Economic importance of plant diseases

Farmers lose a considerable portion of income as their crops and produce are attacked by various insects, diseases and weeds leading to a significant reduction in crop productivity and lower actual yield than the attainable yield of crops. Food crops must compete with 30,000 species of weeds, 3,000 species of nematodes and 10,000 species of plant-eating insects. Yield losses caused by pests, pathogens, and weeds are responsible for 20–40% loss of global agricultural productivity. In India, 20-25% crop losses are reported due to pest attacks every year. As per the estimate by the Central pollution Board of the Govt. of India, the highest food grain loss is due to weed (28%), by diseases (25%), by insects (23%), during storage (10%), by rats (8%), and by others (6%). If we consider , on an average , crop loss of 20%, and the present gross value of our agriculture produce as Rs. 7 lakh crores, the loss comes to Rs. 1, 40,000 crore, which is huge. Even if we could save 50% by using plant protection chemicals, it will add 70, 000 crores additional income to our farmers. At a time, when all of us concerned about National Food Security, can the country afford these losses. Some classical examples of plant diseases that have caused severe losses in the past are shown in Table below.

Classical examples of severe losses caused by plant diseases

Sl.No	Major disease outbreaks	Causal Organism	Year	Location	Comments
1	Late blight of potato	*Phytophthora infestans*	1845–1846	Cool, humid climates	Irish Famine
2	Coffee rust	*Hemileia vastatrix*	1870s–1880s	Asia, South America	Destroyed all coffee in southeast Asia
3	Brown spot of rice	*Drechslera oryzae*	1943	Asia	Bengal famine
4	Downy mildew of grapes	*Plasmopara viticola*	1870s–1880s	U.S., Europe	European epidemic

Recently, India fought a battle against desert locusts whose attack had wiped out lush green fields laden with crops like bajra, sorghum; maize, green gram, black gram, castor, wheat, cotton and vegetable crops spread over 50,000 hectares in Rajasthan, Gujarat, Madhya Pradesh, Uttar Pradesh, Punjab and Maharashtra. The use of insecticide Malathion helped very effectively in managing the situation. Plant protection chemicals are help in preventing rats, mice, flies and other insects from contaminating the food whilst in storage.The major importance of plant diseases are summarized here

1. Limit the kinds of plants and industries in the area.
2. Reduce the quality and quantity of plant produce.
3. May make plants poisonous to humans and animals.
4. May cause financial losses.
5. Cost of controlling plant diseases is also a direct loss to diseases.

Categories of plant diseases

There are number of diseases which attacks crop plants. Therefore It is mandatory to classify plant disease into more manageable and more specific group based on several criteria for easy and better understanding. Let us discuss one by one.

1. On the basis of type of infection

On the basis of type of infection disease can be classified into two types

i. **Localized disease**- Affecting only a part of the plant; leaf spots and anthracnoses.
ii. **Systemic disease**-Affecting the entire plant like mosaic and leaf curl disease.

2. Based on their occurrence

Based on their occurrence the disease can be divided into four groups:

1. **Endemic disease**: When a disease is more or less constantly present in one form or other or less constantly present form year to year in a moderate to

severe form, in a particular country or part of earth, it is classed as endemic. Ex. Wart disease of potato in Darjelling districts.

2. **Epidemic or epiphytotic diseases**: The term 'epidemic' means 'among the people' and in true sense applies to those diseases of human beings which appear very virulently among large section of the population.

   To carry the same sense in the case of plant diseases, the term **epiphytotic** has been coined. An epiphytotic disease is one which occurs widely but periodically. It may be present constantly in the locality but assumes severe form only on occasions. Ex. Irish famine due to late blight of potato

3. **Sporadic diseases**: Sporadic diseases are those diseases which occur at very irregular intervals and locations and in relatively few instances. Ex. Potato spindle tuber,

4. **Pandemic diseases**: When a disease is prevalent throughout the country, continent or the world it is known as a *pandemic* disease. Latest example corona disease.

3. Based on the cause

Based on the cause the disease can be divided into two parts

1. **Infectious or Biotic disease:**These are diseases incited by biotic or mesobiotic agents under a set of suitable environments. Example, fungal disease, bacterial disease, viral disease.

2. **Non-infectious or Abiotic disease:** These are the diseases with no biotic or mesobiotic agents associated, remain noninfectious and cannot be transmitted from one diseased plant to another healthy plant. Example. Disease caused by nature-frost, rain, wind, sun, hail storm

4. Based on the production of inoculum

Based on the production of inoculum, the disease can also be divided into two parts;

1. **Single cycle disease (Simple interest disease):** When the increase of disease is mathematically analogs to simple interest of money, it is called simple interest disease. There is only one generation of disease in the course of one epidemic. Such diseases develop from a common source of inoculums i.e the capital i.e inoculum is constant. Example. Loose smut of wheat.

2. **Multiple cycle disease (Compound interest disease):** When the increase in disease is mathematically analogues to compound interest of money, the disease is called compound interest disease. There are several or many generations of the pathogen in one life cycle of the crop. The capital ie inoculum is increased by the amount of interest. Example. Late blight of potato.

5. On the basis of type of perpetuation and spread

On the basis of type of perpetuation and spread, the disease can be divided into three groups

1. **Soil-borne diseases**: The causal agents perpetuate and spread through soil. Example. Damping off and Fusarium wilt
2. **Seed-borne diseases**: Seed or seed materials help in the perpetuation and spread of this disease. The disease causing agents may be internally seed-borne or externally seed-borne .Example: Loose smut of wheat (Example of internally seed borne), Blast of rice (Example of externally seed-borne).
3. **Air-borne diseases**: In these type of diseases the causal agents are spread by wind (air). Example. Early leaf spot and late leaf spot of groundnut c.

6. Based on symptoms

Based on symptoms the disease can be classified into rusts smuts, wilts, blights, cankers, mildews, rots, damping-off, die-back, scab etc.

7. Based on the host plant

On the basis of host diseases are classified like disease of apple, diseases of wheat, diseases of rose, diseases of coconut, diseases of coffee, diseases of cotton.

8. Based on sugar requirement of the pathogen

Based on the sugar requirements of the pathogen, diseases can be grouped into high sugar diseases or low sugar diseases. Diseases such as rusts and powdery mildews increased when the crops were sprayed with chemicals like DDT or maleic hydrazide which inhibit the outflow of sugars from the leaf and termed these diseases as 'high sugar diseases'. On the other hand when the crops were sprayed with chemicals like 2,4 D which increase the outflow of sugars e.g. the disease like spots increased and termed these diseases as 'low sugar diseases'

3

Integrated Disease Management (IDM): Introduction, Definition, Concepts, Importance and Objectives of Integrated Disease Management

Origin of the concept of Integrated Control

With some important exceptions, applied plant pathology was for many years rather single minded. It aimed at eradication or total exclusion of a plant disease , and it relied largely on a single control method, application of chemical poisons.

Plant pathologists found an effective and cheap fungicide, so cheap it could often be applied without regard to economic thresholds. With time it was discovered that chemicals caused serious repercussions in the ecosystem. Among the effects were the emergence of resistant strains and the emergence of treated populations, outbreaks of formerly secondary pathogens , population reductions of bioagents, and concatenated effects on other animals, including man-the whole matter of residues, hazards and legal complications. It was also seen that either time the costs of adequate control rose, now often exceeding economically permissible levels.

In the last decades, a revolution in thinking and strategies has occurred. Advances had been made in disease management in crop, where logistics and economic usually prohibit chemical treatment. From this and other work came two developments. One was biological control and other was the concept of maintenance of disease to tolerable economic levels.

As a result, a broader concept of control began in the 1950s . It was called integrated control. Integrated control is defined as a disease management system that , in context of the associated environment and the population dynamics of the pathogen, utilizes all suitable techniques and methods in as compatible a manner as possible and maintains the disease level at levels below those causing economic injury. In a more common sense, it applies to the coordinated management of all pathogen populations in the agricultural environment. It is not simply the superimposition of two control techniques but the integration of all suitable management techniques with the natural regulating and limiting elements of the environment.

Impact of book "Silent Springs"

The publication of classic book Silent Springs by Rachel Carson essentially brought two issues into sharp focus

a) Chemical pesticides can be dangerous to human being as well as the environment and should be used as the last resort.\

b) There are biologically based more safe alternatives to synthetic pesticides and these eco-friendly methods need to be studied and exploited.

The message of Carlson and indiscriminate use of pesticides make policy maker seriously concerned. Therefore, the policy adopted by the World Bank since 1980s is to finance projects that donot seriously compromise on public health or cause irreversible environmental deterioration. The World Bank objective is focused on the IPM approach for sustainable agriculture.

What is Integrated Disease Management?

The Integrated disease management consists of three words

- Integrated
- Disease
- Management

Integrated

- Means that a broad interdisciplinary approach is taken using scientific principles of crop protection to combine into a single cropping system a variety of management strategies and tactics to reduce disease.
- **Strategies** are the general approaches used to implement coordinated systems of multiple tactics. Examples are containment, preventive, corrective or remedial, and eradication.
- **Tactics** are the specific methods used to achieve pest control. These include cultural, biological, physical, genetic, chemical, and regulatory procedures.

Disease

- Disease (literally dis-ease) implies lack of 'comfort' and therefore , involves deviation from normal functioning.
- Disease as a malfunctioning process involving more or less continuous interaction between host and pathogen occurring through a large number of quantitative changes between qualitative states of healthy and diseased conditions.

Management

- Implies a process by which information is collected and used to make good management decisions to reduce losses from disease in a planned, coordinated way.

- IDM requires a more tolerant management approach than traditional pesticide-based programs.
- Eradicating all diseases from a crop is the not the objective .
- IDM emphasizes disease suppression rather than eradication.

Integrated Disease management (IDM) - a Smart, Sensible and Sustainable approach to disease control:

- **Smart** : Because IDM creates a safer and healthier learning environment by managing diseases and reducing exposure to pests and pesticides.
- **Sensible:** Since practical strategies are used to reduce sources of food, water and shelter for pests .
- **Sustainable:** Because the emphasis is on prevention, which makes it an economically advantageous approach.

Definitions

"Selection, integration, and implementation of disease control based on predicted economic, ecological, and sociological consequences".

"A comprehensive approach to disease control that uses combined means to reduce the status of disease to tolerable levels while maintaining a quality environment".

"The optimization of disease control in an economically and ecologically sound manner, accomplished by the coordinated use of multiple tactics to assure stable crop production and to maintain disease loss below the economic injury level while minimizing risks to man and the environment".

"A sustainable approach to manage diseases by combining biological, cultural, physical and chemical tools in a way that minimizes economic, health and environmental risks".

"The careful consideration of all available disease control techniques and subsequent integration of appropriate measures that discourage the development of diseases and keep pesticides and other interventions to levels that are economically justified and reduce or minimize risks to human health and the environment. IDM emphasizes the growth of a healthy crop with the least possible disruption to agro-ecosystems and encourages natural disease control mechanisms".

Concept of IDM

This definition incorporates the underlying concepts that:

- IDM is not a "package" but is location specific.
- IDM is a combination of all suitable techniques.
- IDM is farmer based.
- IDM must be considered as an integral part of integrated crop management.
- IDM considers the economics of disease management.
- IDM optimizes pesticide use.

- IDM promotes safe handling and application for the protection of health and the environment – as little as possible, as much as necessary.

1. IDM is not a package of fixed recommendations

- There is no single "recipe" for IDM.
- Even within one crop, there will be differences between locations, crop growth, yield potential, the attacks of the different diseases and the farmer's resources.
- It is impossible to give one package of recommendations that will adequately cope with all the combinations of these possibilities.
- The implementation of IDM, therefore, must be flexible, and adapt to local agronomic, disease, and farmer circumstances.

2. IDM is a combination of all suitable techniques

- IDM is a combination of all suitable technique which minimize disease level and damage.
- The actual techniques included in an IDM programme will vary, not only between crops, but also within the same crop grown in different locations, depending on the suitability of the different techniques for that situation and availability of tools and resources.

3. IDM is farmer based

- As the farmer is the one who has to put the techniques into practice in his or her field.
- The farmer must, therefore, possess the knowledge and the resources required to do this.

4. IDM must be considered as an integral part of crop production

- Pest management cannot be considered on its own, it is a part of the overall production practice of a crop, which include seed/variety selection, land preparation, fertility and water management etc.
- Changes to production practices will affect pest management practices.

5. IDM considers the economics of disease management

- IDM must be considered as an integral part of crop production together with all integrated crop management (ICM).
- Disease management cannot be considered on its own, it is a part of the overall production practice of a crop.
- Changes to production practices will affect pest management practices.

6. IDM considers the economics of disease management

- IDM considers the economics of disease management as the crop has to pay for all the input costs.

- If unnecessary inputs such as unnecessary pesticide applications are used , profits and the farmer's income are reduced.

7. IDM optimizes pesticide use

- IDM eliminates unnecessary use of pesticide.
- It promotes safe handling and application for the protection of health and the environment – as little as possible, as much as necessary.

Why is IDM Important?

The demand of a growing population for food and fiber require farmers to produce more crops on existing farmland. To increase these yields requires continuous improvement of agricultural technologies to minimize crop losses. The challenge is to do this while protecting the environment. IDM is a big part of the solution. Increasingly it is being adopted in India for long-term, sustainable agriculture that achieves adequate, safe and quality food production, improves farmer livelihoods and conserves non-renewable resources.

General principles for using an IDM programme

The following are general principles for using an integrated disease management in the design of programmes for sustainable agriculture.

- Any disease exists at some tolerable level: Any disease exists at some tolerable level – this notion forms the basis of the economic injury level concept.
- Use an ecosystem approach to anticipate potential disease problems associated with intensified crop production. The production system should use, for example, a diverse range of disease-resistant crop varieties, crop rotations, intercropping, optimized planting time and weed management. To reduce losses, control strategies should take advantage of biocontrol agents, along with biopesticides and selective, low risk synthetic pesticides. Investment will be needed in strengthening farmers' knowledge and skills.
- Undertake contingency planning for when credible evidence of a significant disease threat emerges. That will require investment in seed systems to support deployment of resistant varieties, and crop-free periods to prevent the carryover of pathogen populations to the following season. Selective pesticides with adequate regulatory supervision will need to be identified, and specific communication campaigns prepared.
- Analyse the nature of the cause of disease outbreaks when problems occur, and develop strategies accordingly. Problems may be caused by a combination of factors– for example, summer ploughing that suppresses pathogen surviving in the soil. In the case of seed borne diseases like loose smut of wheat, methods of biological or chemical seed treatment used in the place of soil treatment .
- Determine how much production is at risk, in order to establish the appropriate scale of disease control campaigns or activities. Infestation (not loss) of more

than 10 percent of a crop area is an outbreak that demands a rapid policy response. However, risks from diseases are often over-estimated, and crops can to some extent compensate physiologically for disease damage. The response should not be disproportionate.

- Undertake surveillance to track disease patterns in real time, and adjust response. Geo referenced systems for plant disease surveillance use data from fixed plots, along with roving survey data and mapping and analysis tools.
- Management unit is the agro ecosystem : The management unit is the agro ecosystem and any management action may produce unexpected and undesirable effects – this notion forms the basis of the systems or holistic approach to IDM.

Objectives of IDM

The basic objectives of any IDM program should be to achieve at least the following:

- Reduce the possibility of introducing diseases into the crop.
- Avoid creating conditions suitable for disease establishment and spread.
- Simultaneous management of multiple pathogens.
- Regular monitoring of pathogen effects, and their natural enemies and antagonists as well.
- Use of economic or treatment thresholds when applying chemicals.
- Integrated use of multiple, suppressive tactics.

Goals of an IDM program

- Optimize profits.
- Sustain resource.
- Rational use of pesticides.
- Reduce environmental contamination and costs.
- Utilize natural biological controls.
- Minimize pesticide resistance problems.
- Minimize pest resurgence and secondary pest outbreaks.
- Food safety.
- Worker safety.

Integrated disease management philosophy

1. Recognizes there is no "cure-all" in disease control

- IDM is a philosophy. That is, we recognize that there are no cure-alls and easy methods to manage diseases.
- Reliance on a single tactic will favor diseases that are resistant to that practice.

2. Determine and correct the cause of the disease problem.

- IDM stresses reliance on preventive practices and balances the strengths of one practice against the weaknesses of another to provide a holistic disease management approach.
- Rescue or curative treatments are used only if the preventive practices fail.
- For example, a preventive practice might be planting a yellow mosaic virus resistant/tolerant soybean variety. Only when whitefly populations are above economic threshold level, will an insecticide treatment may be obligatory. Hopefully, by planting the YMV resistant variety you might not spray for YMV during most kharif season.

3. Eradication of a disease is seldom required or even desirable, and is generally not even possible.

- IDM realizes that some disease loss is acceptable.
- Focus should be on economics before management techniques implemented.
- Rescue treatments should only be initiated when the cost of control is less that the amount of loss expected.

4. IDM is a continuum that will change with time.

- Every farmer practices some type of IDM.
- Some are just further along than others. But as long as they make progress to better management that's fine.
- As new disease management techniques are discovered, the producer and crop advisor must adapt their disease management program to reflect these changes.
- What is considered a good IDM program today, may be considered a chemical intensive program in a few years.
- Producer and crop advisor is advised to try innovative changes first on a limited scale, becoming comfortable with the suggested practices before wide-scale changes.

5. Pesticides can to be used in an IDM program only as a last resort and of course in a manner that is legal

- Pesticides are a part of an IDM Program.
- They are a very important part in some cropping systems.
- Some diseases because of sheer percentage, continuous occurrence, low thresholds or because of food contamination issues dictate pesticide use.
- However, pesticides should only be used as a last resort and only when all other management techniques, including preventative techniques, have failed or are no longer economical.
- They also must be used in a manner that is legal (rate, application type, target crop, target pest, etc.).

Criteria of Priority

The FAO of the United Nations has been interested in developing integrated pest/ disease management since 1963 and has developed and implemented several field projects in different parts of the world. This organization recommended for global programme to be undertaken on the basis of programmed priority. Criteria of programme priority have ben asccrtained that point out the necessity of IPM/IDM. These criteria are the following.

- Crop must be of vital national and regional importance .
- Economic /Serious losses are caused by diseases.
- Inadequate control by use of organic pesticides.
- Use of pesticide is generating more problem, but the same cannot be given up otherwise food production will not be stepped up.
- An integrated approach can be developed , which will yield desirable results and be acceptable to growers.

Advantages of IDM

Some of the advantages of an integrated approach are as follows:

- Stable, reliable and quality crop yields.
- Decreased severity of diseases.
- Reduced potential for problems of pest resistance or resurgence.
- Increased consumer confidence in the safety and quality of food and fiber products.
- Improved crop profitability.
- Appropriate use of crop protection products.
- Sustained market share and access of crop protection industry.
- New opportunities for established and novel products, techniques and services.
- Longer product life cycles.
- Increased public confidence in, and credibility of, the crop protection industry.

Disadvantages of IDM

- IDM requires interdisciplinary approach to solve disease problem. Lack of coordination among different institution is a constraint.
- Research programme based on farmer's need is lacking.
- Pesticide subsidy by Government.
- Lack of information on IDM among farmers and extension worker.

- Lack of training on IDM.
- Some farmers feel it is risky to adopt IDM compared to use of pesticides alone.
- Lack of funds for training farmers and extension workers on the use of IDM.
- Bio-pesticides, bio control agents and other IDM components are not readily available.
- Large farmers discourage small farmers in adopting IDM methods by emphasizing more on their risky and unstable nature.

Implication of IDM

- Simultaneous management of multiple pathogens.
- Regular monitoring of pathogens effects, their natural enemies and antagonists as well.
- Use of economic or treatment threshold when applying chemicals.
- Integrated use of multiple and suppressive tactics

Professional Disease Management

1. Professional disease Management is equipping farmers with digital tools to help them best monitor their fields and before any particular problem could cause harm.
2. These digital tools help provide PEACE OF MIND to our farmers.
3. It shifts mindsets to be PREVENTATIVE rather than CURATIVE .
4. Equips farmers with the CONFIDENCE to stay ahead of any challenges.
5. This has proved hugely beneficial to farmers and extension officers in recent months of the corona pandemic.
6. These preventative measures and innovative digital tools have enabled farmers to do the important work of keeping public spaces and crop free of pests even during the shutdown.
7. Moving forward, digital tools and innovative solutions will continue to be driving forces in the pursuit of keeping our environments – and our crop -- free from pests in a sustainable way.

4

Methods of Detection and Diagnosis of Diseases

Detection/Diagnosis

Detection

1. Detection means the existence of whatever do you want detecting but diagnosis is that the analysis in depth of existing thing.
2. Objectively look for, listen to the credible complains, symptoms that is sometimes not visible at all .
3. It is art or skill of identifying some abnormalities, i.e. which is below or higher than the normal permissible range/threshold.

Diagnosis

1. It means to ascertain the specific medical condition that is causing the problem.
2. It a complex problem, where based on known theory, physiology, pathological findings, his experience one has to come to conclusion and answer to the question that "Why such symptoms exist? "
3. It is a-priory step for prescribing medications for the plants.

Diagnosis of plant disease

Diagnosis of plant disease is to identify the disease nature and to determine the causal agent whether living or nonliving.

How does a plant pathologist go about diagnosing plant problems?

1. Diagnostician must have very good observation skills.
2. Needs to be a good detective.
3. Keep an open mind until all of the facts related to the problem can be collected.
4. Possibility of multiple causal factors must also be considered.
5. Control measures depend on proper identification of diseases and of the causal agents.
6. Without proper identification of the disease and the disease causing agent, disease control measures can be a waste of time and money and can lead to further plant losses.
7. Proper disease diagnosis is therefore vital

Techniques used for detection of pathogens

1. **Conventional**: On the basis of recognising symptoms, growth in culture, microscopy .
2. **Serological**: Interaction between antigen and antibody.
3. **Molecular techniques**: Nucleic acid based methods.

1. Conventional

1. Recognising symptoms
2. Growth in culture
3. Microscopy
4. Staining

Recognising symptoms

1. Symptoms of disease in infected plants can help us diagnose which pathogen is responsible.
2. Different pathogens can cause similar symptoms.
3. Ooze production is the characteristic symptoms of plant pathogenic bacteria.
4. It's usually necessary to do further diagnostic tests to accurately identify the pathogen causing the disease

Advantages

1. Quick when symptoms are distinct.

Disadvantages

1. Symptoms must clearly confirm to a well known syndrome.
2. Soil obscures symptoms.
3. Requires much prior knowledge on the part of the inspector.

Growth in culture

1. Testing often starts by taking a sample from plant tissue showing symptoms of infection.
2. Cells from the sample are spread over a Petri dish that contains a growth medium such as PDA.
3. Growth medium contains nutrients.
4. Petri dish is kept in warm conditions in an incubator.
5. Bacteria and fungi from the sample grow to form cultures.
6. Appearance of a culture, such as its colour and furriness, can help a pathologist to identify the pathogen.

7. Different substances can be added to the growth medium to encourage or inhibit the growth of particular microorganisms.
8. This can help to identify the pathogens present in the sample.
9. Ex. *Xanthonas axonopodis pv. citri* gives yellowish color growth when streaked on growth media.
10. Ex. In fungi; Rhizopus species gives the cottony growth on PDA while, *Geotrichum candidum* gives the condensed growth.

Advantages

1. Assesses living (culturable) microbes.
2. Able to recognize viable cells in a sample.
3. Easy to quantitate cells in a sample.
4. High sensitivity with appropriate media.

Disadvantages

1. Identification is not always straightforward.
2. High skill level is necessary for optimal results.
3. Specific growth media may be lacking.
4. Time and resource intensive.
5. Risk of contamination.
6. Relies on phenotypic biochemical characterization.

Microscopy

1. Microsocpy detect the pathogen on the basis of morphology.
2. Bacteria, fungi and protists(but not viruses) can usually be observed using a light microscope.
3. Different pathogens have different shapes.
4. Some pathogens grow in pairs or chains. These characteristics can help us to identify them.
5. Different pathogens can be stained different colours using dyes.
6. One commonly used dye is Gram stain. This is another piece of evidence that can help us to identify them.
7. In case of fungi; reproductive structures, spore can be seen under microscope.
8. From which you can identify fungus up to genera level.
9. Nematodes can be detected after preparing slide from suspension, and visualized it under microscope.

Advantages

1. Easy to operate.
2. Do not take up much space in the laboratory.
3. Easily transportable.
4. Non-perturbing.
5. Non expensive (Exception electron microscope).
6. Viruses and bacteria can be examined by electron microscopy.

Disadvantages

1. Requires careful expert inspection.
2. Microscopy is expensive.
3. Inability to operate in darkness.
4. Low resolution.
5. Inability to provide a 3D rendering of structures.
6. Electron microscopy requires expertise.
7. Lack of diagnostic stains for fungi.

Staining

1. Bacterial cells, fungi and nematode can be colored with a stain.
2. Provide contrast with the background to make cellular organalles visible.
3. Simple staining; methylene blue, basic fushchin and crystal violet.
4. Steps for staining bacterial smear.
    - Pass the slide, smear the slide up through a flame three times.
    - Flood the smear with a stain and let stand one minute.
    - Rinse the slide gently with water, making sure the stream of water does not strike the smear directly.

Gram staining

- Developed in 1884 by Danish physician Hans Christian Gram.
- Corner stone of bacterial identification and the taxonomic division.
- Scientific technique of staining that is used to differentiate the species of bacteria into 2 main groups, namely the gram-positive and the gram-negative bacteria.
- The differences between these groups of bacteria are considered to be important in determining appropriate treatments for infections.

Advantages

1. It gives quick results when examining infections.
2. It is simple and cost-effective.

3. It helps with determining appropriate treatments for infection.
4. It is basically a key procedure in identifying bacteria.

Disadvantages

1. It has significant limitations when used for environmental microbiology.
2. It has a few side effects.
3. It comes with certain types of risks.
4. It might lead to misinterpretation.

2. Serological techniques

A method using the specificity of the antigen antibody reaction for the detection and identification of antigenic substances and the organism that carry them

1. Based on the specificity of antigen-antibody reactions.
2. Used for the diagnosis of plant viruses for many years.
3. Of late, these techniques have also been applied to diagnose fungi, bacteria and phytoplasmas.
4. Techniques originally based on the use of polyclonal antibodies (a mixture antibody), which often reduced the reliability of the test due to nonspecific cross reactions.
5. Development of monoclonal antibodies, which have narrow specificity against a single type of antigen, has greatly improved the accuracy of such tests.
6. Polyclonal antibody often react with several species within a genus, where as monoclonal antibodies discriminate between different species within the genus.
7. A sample from an infected plant can be put on a test strip that is coated with monoclonal antibodies.The antibodies recognize an antigen from a specific pathogen.
8. Test strip works like a home pregnancy test. The test line on the strip will change colour when the antigen from the pathogen is present

Use of Serological techniques

1. To determine relationships between viruses.
2. To identify a virus causing plant disease.
3. To detect virus in foundation stocks of plants.
4. To detect symptomless viral infection.
5. To measure virus quantitatively.
6. To locate the virus within a cell or tissue.
7. To detect plant viruses in insects and to purify a virus.

Advantages

1. Must are simple techniques that require little expertise.
2. Most methods are quick.
3. An accurate result may be obtained.
4. Pathogens which cause diseases with variable or latent symptoms on the host plant can be separated.
5. Pathogens with an indistinct structure or an undistinguished morphology, such as in many groups of viruses and bacteria, may be distinguished.
6. A number of commercial kits are available.
7. There is an almost unlimited potential for more kits to be produced.
8. Specificity to a particular strain, species, genus or any other taxonmay be chosen.

Disadvantages

1. Animal handling is still necessary requiring expertise despite development of *in vitro* systems.
2. Specific methods have not yet been developed for most diseases.
3. In general too many antigens occur in common between fungi and plants to permit the use of polyclonal antibodies to diagnose fungi in host tissues even when unwanted cross reactions have been reduced by using pure antigen.
4. Not effective for viruses that lack a protein or related component, against which to raise an antibody.
5. Only a few percent of hybridoma cell lines can be expected to produce valuable monoclonal antibodies.
6. High capital cost of fusion.
7. High initial costs of raising and selecting specific monoclonal antibodies.

Types of serological tests

1. Precipitin test
2. Gel diffusion test
3. Agglutination reaction
4. Elisa (Direct and Indirect)

1. Precipitin test

- Earliest and quite common method.
- Antigen and antibody are mixed in a solution.

2. Gel diffusion test

- Antigen & Antibody diffuse toward one another through agar gel and meet in a zone in suitable concentrations.

3. Agglutination reaction

- When antigen is adsorbed on the surface of a large particle such as cell, plastid etc and these are precipitated by addition of antibodies.
- In all these tests the reaction of antigen and antibody becomes visible either by precipitation of the two on the bottom of the test tube or by formation of a band at the interface where the two meet.

4. Enzyme-Linked ImmunosorbentAssay (ELISA)

1. Molecular method for identification of diseases based on antibodies and color change in the assay.
2. In this method, the target antigens from the viruses, bacteria and fungi are made to specifically bind with antibodies conjugated to an enzyme.
3. The detection can be visualized based on color changes resulting from the interaction between the substrate and the immobilized enzyme.
4. Performance of ELISA can be improved greatly with the application of specific monoclonal and recombinant antibodies which are commercially available .
5. Specific monoclonal antibodies have been used in ELISA to achieve lower limits of detection in the order of 10^5–10^6 CFU/mL.
6. For plant disease detection, tissue print-ELISA and lateral flow devices that enable detection have been fabricated for on-site detection.
7. However, the sensitivity for bacteria is relatively low (10^5–10^6 CFU/mL, making it useful only for the confirmation of plant.

Two types

1. Direct ELISA
2. IndirectELISA

1. Direct ELISA (Double antibody sandwich ELISA)

- The wells (capacity 0.4 ml) of a polystyrene microtiterplate are first filled with and then emptied of, sequentially,
  a. Antibodies to the virus.
  b. Virus preparation or sap from an infected plant.
  c. Antibodies to the virus to which molecules of a particular enzyme have been attached.
  d. A substrate for the enzyme , that is , a substance that the enzyme can break down and cause change in its color.
- The substrate is not emptied but is kept in the well.
- Within 30 or 60 minutes, the wells are read either visually or preferably with a colorimeter that measures the amount of color in each well.

- Presence of color in the well indicates that there was virus in the sample (step b above).
- Degree of visible coloration or the size of the reading given by the colorimeter is proportional to and therefore a measure of the amount of virus present in the sample.

2. Indirect ELISA

- Sequence of steps b and a is reversed.
- The wells (capacity 0.4 ml) of a polystyrene microtiterplate are first filled with and then emptied of, sequentially.
  - a) Virus preparation or sap from an infected plant.
  - b) Antibodies to the virus.
  - c) Antibodies in the antibody-enzyme complex are not those against the virus, they are antibodies against the antibody proteins of the animal in which the virus antibody are produced.(They are anti-rabbit antibodies produced in still in another animal, such as goat).

Advantages of indirect ELISA

- The same goat anti rabbit antibody enzyme complex can be used in steps c for assays for any virus, as long as the first antibodies , that is those against the virus used in step b, were produced in rabbit.

Serology of plant viruses

1. Antigen: A virus protein or any other foreign protein .
2. When antigen injected into a mammal (rabbit, mouse, horse) orbird (chicken,turkey), it induces animal to produce specific new protein called Antibodies.
3. Antibodies circulate in the blood fluid or serum of animal.
4. Antibodies react specifically with and bind to a small portion of the surface called Antigenic determinant of the antigen injected.
5. Each antigen has many different antigenic determinants site surface and produces antiserum.
6. An antigen producing cell is fused with a mouse myeloma(cell) ,it produces a hybrid cell that can grow in culture indefinitely and continues to produce monoclonal antibodies for a long time.
7. Such antibody producing hybrid cell is called hybridomas.
8. Hybridomas can be grown in culture for months or years and produce large quantities of identical monoclonal antibodies.

Monoclonal Vs Polyclonal antibodies

Sl.No	Monoclonal	Polyclonal
1	Antiserum contain single antibody	Antiserum contains a mixture of different antibodies.
2	Each antibody react only with single antigen of pathogen	Each antibody reacting with the antigen but at a different surface locality.

3. Molecular Technique

Any properties of an individual's showing heritable variations is referred to as a character.

These characters which can be easily identified are referred to as marker.

Types of markers

Sl.No	Name of marker		Remarks
1	Morphological Markers	•	Markers related to size, color, and surface of the various parts.
		•	Such characters are used for varietal identifications
2	Biochemical Markers	•	Markers related to variations in protein and amino acids banding patterns.
		•	Gel electrophoresis studies are used for identification of biochemical markers.
3	Molecular markers	•	An unique sequence of nucleotides found on a strand of DNA.
		•	Markers related to variations in DNA fragments generated by restriction endonuclease enzymes.
		•	DNA markers are also used at molecular markers.
		•	Also called genetic markers or DNA markers.

Polymerase Chain Reaction (PCR)

1. Also called molecular photocopying.
2. PCR technique was invented by Kary *B. Mullis* in 1985.
3. It is a molecular biology technique for enzymatically replicating DNA without using living organisms like *E.coli*, Yeast.
4. PCR are used to amplify or make many copies of small fragment of DNA.
5. PCR process is directed by a machine called thermocycler.
6. The machine is programmed to alter the temperature of the reaction every few minutes to allow DNA denaturing and synthesis.
7. Taq polymerase enzyme, which is tolerant to high temperature is used in the PCR process.
8. Taq polymerase was discovered in hot springs from the bacteria *Thermus auquaticus*.

9. DNA polymerase is stable at high temperatures needed to perform the amplification.

Procedure of PCR

Each cycle of PCR consists of three important steps.

Denaturing

1. Achieved at high temperature (94-96^{0}C).
2. Makes both templates DNA primers single stranded.
3. Takes usually 1-2 minutes.

Annealing

1. Achieved by lowering the temperature (45-60^{0}C).
2. Leads to attachment of primers (single stranded) to single DNA strands.

Elongation

1. Allows DNA polymerase to copy to DNA strand.
2. Final elongation step is used after the last cycle.

Application

1. Repeated heating and cooling cycles make several copies of the target DNA.
2. Twenty PCR cycles can be completed and millions of copies of the target DNA can be made in about one hour.
3. PCR was initially used for highly specific detection of diseases caused by fungi, bacteria and viruses, viroids, mycoplasma etc.
4. Reverse-transcription PCR (RT-PCR) has also been used for plant pathogen identification due to its high sensitivity.
5. Multiplex PCR was proposed to enable simultaneous detection of different DNA or RNA by running a single reaction .
6. Real-time PCR platforms have also been used for on-site, rapid diagnosis of plant diseases based on the bacterial, fungal and viral nucleic acids.

Advantages of PCR

1. Fast and inexpensive techniques.
2. It permits amplification of the targeted segment of DNA.
3. Used to clone gene of interest.
4. Performed with small amount of DNA.
5. *In vitro* multiplication of DNA.
6. Widely used by researchers.

PCR based method for detection of plant pathogen

1. Conventional PCR
2. Nested PCR
3. Multiplex PCR
4. Reverse Transcription-PCR
5. Real time PCR

1. Conventional PCR

1. Basic method for the identification of fungal pathogens at different taxonomic levels i.e. genus, species or strain, depending on the specificity of the primers.
2. Identified *Sclerotium rolfsii* by conventional PCR method and developed *Colletotrichum capsici*, based in specific sequence of internal transcribed spacer (ITS) region.

Nested PCR

1. Nested PCR is a variation of the polymerase chain reaction, in that two pairs (in stead of one pair) of PCR primers are used to amplify a fragment.
2. First pair of PCR primer amplify a fragment similar to a standard PCR.
3. Second pair of primers called nested primers bind in side the first PCR product fragment to allow amplification of a second PCR product which is shorter than the first one.
4. This method has been widely used for detection and characterization of numerous fungi.

Multiplex PCR

1. Multiplex PCR approach is used when more than two primer involve in the same reaction allowing the simultaneous and sensitive detection of different DNA targets.
2. This approach is highly useful for the identification of plant pathology since plants are usually infected by more than one pathogen.
3. This PCR has been used for the simultaneous detection and differentiation of *Podosphaera xanthii* and *Golovinomyces cichoracearum* in sunflower, for detecting *Phytophthora lateralis* in cedar trees and water samples, including detection of an internal control in the same reaction.

Reverse Transcription-PCR

1. This approach can be used to amplify RNA sequence in DNA duplex.
2. In this technique, cDNA copy of the RNA is produced using the enzyme reverse transcriptase.
3. This cDNA is then used for amplification.

4. m-RNA is degraded rapidly in dead cells, the detection of mRNA by RT-PCR is considered an accurate indicator of cell viability.
5. RT-PCR has been used to detect viable population of *Mycosphaerella graminicola* in wheat.
6. This approaches highly valuable in phyto- pathology for the analysis of fungal gene expression during disease development.

Real time PCR

1. RT PCR is the most sensitive method and can discriminate between closely related mRNAs.
2. Developed to quantitate differences in m RNA production, particularly in such cases where only small amounts of cells/tissue are available.
3. The various methods of mRNA quantitation include northern hybridization, ribonuclease protection assays, situ hybridization, and RT-PCR.
4. Conventional PCR does not yield truly and accurate quantitative result because ethidium bromide does not give a bright fluorescence, and when a band is detectable the logarithmic phase of amplification is already over.
5. Real time PCR is capable to perform multiplex detection of two or more pathogens in the same reaction.

5

Economic Thresholds and Injury Levels

Keys to Disease Management

- Disease management and pest management are parts of crop management, but they demand a specific expertise.
- Disease management is the sum total of all actions, intentional , or not, that serve to regulate disease levels so that they remain below the economic threshold level.
- The action can be directed towards a single disease or toward all diseases threatening a crop.
- Development of disease management program depends on knowledge of three areas; crop economics , population dynamics and disease control technology.
- Economic considerations are crucial in the process leading to a decision for or against disease. Economic thresholds and Injury Levels play a important role.

Disease Management and Decision Making

Decisions need to be taken by the farmer as to how to implement disease management in the most effective and economic manner. Many of these decisions are taken a long time before any diseases appear, such as the crop rotation, time of planting, amount of fertiliser, etc. During the growing season, however, continual decisions need to be made regarding disease management. The disease management decision making process is a continuous cycle that can be summarized as:

1. Detection

- Continual monitoring to see what disease and natural enemies are present in the crop is usually called scouting.
- Diseases are detected before they cause economic loss, and spot treatments can possibly be made.
- If detection is too late, control will be less effective, more costly, and crop losses will occur.

2. Identification

- The organism must be identified to see if it is a disease, a natural enemies, or of no importance.

- If the organism is a disease, it is necessary to identify the stage in the life cycle so that control methods can be directed at the most vulnerable stage.
- For diseases, knowledge of the symptoms is needed for identification.

3. Economic significance

- Is the disease causing, or, if left uncontrolled, will it cause, economic damage or loss?.
- Economic damage is the amount of damage that justifies the costs of control.
- It must be determined, therefore, if the pest numbers or infected areas are high enough to warrant spending money on control. This is usually achieved by treatment thresholds.
- Crop growth stage and economic value also need to be taken into consideration.
- It should be noted that biological damage (for example, holes in leaves) often occurs without there being any yield or economic loss.
- The potential (controlling) impact of beneficial species also needs to be considered.

4. Decision

- If the disease level is below the threshold, then no pesticide treatment should be applied.
- If the disease level is above the threshold, then control treatment is required.

5. Selection of control method(s)

- The method of control must be effective, practical, economic, and safe.
- More than one control method may be involved for a single disease.
- For example the application of a pesticide spray to kill adult mosquitoes and remove the nuisance effect, while at the same time removing breeding sites (draining ponds, cleaning up old tins, bottles, tyres etc that contain water in which the larvae live) to prevent future infestations.

6. Evaluation

- The follow-up of the control method to evaluate the effectiveness.
- This is a continuation of the monitoring procedure at the beginning of the decision making process, and starts the decision making cycle again.

Economic Principles of Disease Management

A farmer grows a crop as a food supply or to make money. In either case, he wants to maximise his yield or profit, and needs to consider both in economic terms.

- Profit = Value of harvested crop – Production costs – Transport/Marketing costs.
- Crop production inputs cost the farmer money. The more he spends on inputs, the less profit he makes.

- All inputs need to be used effectively and economically. In other words, the farmer should only use inputs when they will give an economic or other significant benefit.
- For pesticides, it is the cost over the season that must be considered, not the cost per litre. A pesticide that is cheap per litre may be more expensive over the season as a higher mixing rate may have to be used, or it may be less effective and so require more applications, than a pesticide that is more expensive per litre.
- If disease are at a low level, the value of the crop that will be lost is less than the cost of a pesticide application. In this case, the farmer will lose money by using a pesticide.
- If diseases are at a high level, the value of the crop that will be lost will be greater than the cost of the pesticide application. The use of a pesticide in this case will give a return on the farmers investment in pesticide use.

Economic Thresholds and Injury Levels

- Total eradication of a disease is almost impossible and is usually undesirable because it can spell the end of the disease natural enemies and can upset the natural economic balance.
- It's usually better to determine the level of disease presence or disease related loss you can tolerate without harm to your health and plants.
- Determining these levels or thresholds goes hand and hand with field monitoring and is the back-bone of IDM.

Threshold

A boundary, where something starts or ends.

Importance of thresholds

a. To make decision on scheduling of control and control methods.
b. To establish the optimal amount of control which can be used to minimize risk of economic damage and environmental hazards.

Economic damage

- An amount of injury which will justify the cost of artificial control.

Types of thresholds

Three types

1. Economic Injury Level or Damage Threshold
2. Economic Thresholds orAction Thresholds
3. Warning Threshold

1. Economic Injury Level or Damage Threshold

- The level of disease severity at which the highest economically acceptable damage occurs.
- The lowest population density that will cause economic damage.
- The strategy of disease management is to tolerate disease, but to regulate it at subeconomic levels.
- The level of disease severity at which disease begins to adversely affect yield and or quality- the damage threshold must be know.
- The level of threshold varies with crop, disease and local economy.
- True determination of the damage threshold is part of the fine tuning of local management system and depends not only on biologic information but also on accurate knowledge of the costs of inputs to the system, the value of outputs and the required maintenance level.
- The farmers can afford only that amount of disease control that will produce yield or profit exceeding the cost of the control measures.

2. Economic Thresholds or Action Thresholds

- The density at which control measure should be determined to prevent an increasing disease intensity from reaching the economic injury level.
- The economic threshold is lower than the economic injury level to permit sufficient time for the initiation of disease control measures and for these measures to take effect before the population reaches the economic injury level.
- The rate of disease development depends on host resistance ,pathogen virulence and environmental suitability.
- If initial innoculum, rate of disease development , and the damage threshold are known, it can be predicted at what time disease will exceed the damage threshold.
- If damage threshold (Xd) is known and disease is present, the farmer must know when to act –'the action threshold"
- The farmers must apply a control measure at the right time that will so reduce rate of disease development that disease will not reach the damage threshold before harvest.

4. Warning Threshold

- It is the level of disease severity (Xw) that leads to a standby warning .
- The warning threshold is lower and earlier than the action threshold and the latter is lower and earlier than the damage threshold.
- Mant things have to be done before a farmer can take the appropriate action. The chemical has to be bought , the spray equipment readied, and soon.

How thresholds are developed

Thresholds, mainly used by commercial growers, can be developed from the following factors:

1. Amount of physical damage related to various pest densities; How large the pest population can grow before it causes a certain level of damage.
2. Monetary value and production costs of the crop at various levels of physical damage.
3. Monetary cost of the control measure.
4. History of the field.
5. Determining the danger of the disease or pest at different stages of the crops development.
6. Disease and pest distribution.
7. Monetary loss associated with various levels of physical damage.
8. Amount of physical damage that can be prevented by the control measure.
9. Monetary value of the portion the crop that can be saved by the control measure.
10. How much aesthetic or economic damage can be tolerated?
11. Establish a treatment level that keeps the pest population small enough so it does not cause an unacceptable level of damage.
12. Standard of the end consumer and ultimate destination of the crop,
13. Ability to control the disease and pest rapidly and effectively.

6

Integrated Disease Management (IDM) Tools and Strategies

Integrated disease management includes use of physical, cultural, biological, chemical and biotechnological for disease management. It may comprise computer aided sampling, decision making, improved farm tools & equipment.Farmers are the primary decision makers in Integrated disease management programs. They have to decide individually and collectively how to manage all diseases that may harm crops. The role of researchers and institutions is to provide access to a wide range of suitable technologies, products, services and other possible informations on their optimal use strategies, characteristics and costs specificities.Most farmers will combine diverse IDM tactics and tools.

The prerequisite for development of an Integrated Disease Management program is to understand farmers perceptions of disease problems and their current practices of disease management. IDM recommendations must be flexible enough to adjust to change in the environment, cropping patterns and market focus. The socio-economic effects of IDM components must also be scrutinized. The major IDM strategies and tools are

1. Setting an economic threshold.
2. Protecting natural enemies.
3. Choosing the right products.
4. Using products judiciously and safely.
5. Preventing disease resistance to crop protection products.
6. Role of public and private sector in the widespread adoption of IDM.

1. Setting an economic threshold

- Farmers required simple methods for rapidly determining whether disease level in a crop is likely to cause economic damage.
- It is better to monitor the losses due to disease before deciding to use a crop protection product or other intervention, as the severity of diseases varies.
- Once disease level has reached an economic threshold -it is time to intervene.
- Weather based modeling can indicate the requirement to intervene before the diseases reaches the economic threshold level (eg. Late blight of potato).

- The economic threshold is depending on stage of crop development at which it occurs and on disease level.
- This matters as many crop can compensate for some damage during part of their growth cycle.
- Use of an economic threshold as a decision tool has one difficulty is that it depends on the value of the crop.
- Income from the sale of crops can change quickly based on supply and demand in local markets.
- The severity of disease can be reduced by use of disease resistance varieties, but disease level should still be monitored to see if added intervention is required .
- Practical disease control methods acceptable to farmers need to be develop using local knowledge.
- It is possible in various regions to develop local database to assist in making decisions on an area wide basis.

2. Protecting natural enemies/ biocontrol agents

- Conserving bioagents/ natural enemies of diseases is an important part of IDM and helps to prevent disease resurgence.
- The effect of pesticides or other intervention on both diseases and their biogents need to be considered.
- Population of bioagents can recover relatively quickly, even when broad spectrum products are used and particularly if they are easily degrade.
- It is possible to physically limit the impact of broad spectrum products, part of a crop area can be left untreated to allow bioagents to survive and recolonize the treated areas.
- Timing of application to periods when bioagents are not active need to be considered.

3. Selecting the right products

- Plant protection chemicals that penetrate plant leaves and degrade quickly on leaf surfaces need to be recommended and promoted.
- Plant protection chemicals that may have a minimal impact on non pests also need to be recommended and promoted
- It is crucial to review product characteristics, application & costs etc in developing an IDM program.
- Farmers are required to select the ones that offer the most cost effective treatments with minimal undesirable effects.
- Selective chemicals are less likely to affect bioagents and other non target organisms, need to be promoted.
- Seed treatments are also vital component of IDM program as it protect seedlings from early disease .

- Seed treatments may prevent the need for crop protection products applications later on.

4. Using products responsibly and safely

- Timely and targeted application of crop protection chemicals is key to effective disease management.
- Crop protection chemicals should be used according to manufacturer and scientist's recommendation.
- Prescribed doses should be used to manage diseases and prevent them from developing resistance to products.
- Guidelines on the transport and disposal of unused products, appropriate storage and empty container should also be strictly followed.
- Modest changes in application practices like controlling spray pressure can improve chemical coverage or directing the nozzle to spray where the disease is located on the undersides of leaves and better control diseases.

5. Preventing disease resistance to crop protection chemicals

- IDM offers a different ways to reduce the risk of resistance development.
- Strategies need to be followed to disease resistance from chemicals are scouting, applying pesticides judiciously; rotating different modes of action; restricting the use of single chemical across multiple crops; destroying crop residues; use locally adapted varieties with native resistance etc.
- Continued development of novel active ingredients for crop protection products and new biotech traits would expand the resistance management tools available to farmers.

6. Role of public and private sector in the adoption of IDM

- Development of new products and technologies through innovative research.
- Supporting programs to monitor the effect of the crop protection chemicals on natural enemies and environment.
- Development of IDM skills and understanding among stakeholders.
- Train teaching and technical staff who may teach sales staff, extension officer and farmers about IDM.
- Develop training and education programs for farmers using field schools, mass and social media, newsletters, direct mail, videos and posters.
- Train government & private extension staff, seed distributers and retailers who directly influence farmers and required to be able to provide practical advice about IDM/IPM.

7

Integrated Disease Management (IDM) Components

Integrated disease management (IDM) needs competence in three broad areas

I. Prevention

II. Monitoring

III. Intervention

I. Prevention

- Means prevent the buildup of disease.
- Comprises an array of practical strategies that suit local conditions.

II. Observations/Monitoring

- Monitor crops for both diseases and natural mechanisms.
- Includes scouting for diseases.
- To determine if, when and how intervention should occur.
- Links monitoring with decision making, often together with "expert systems

III. Intervention

- Intervene when management is needed.
- Encompasses physical, cultural, biological, chemical methods to preserve the economic value of crops with minimal effects on the environment.

I. Prevention

- Many aspects of farm and crop management are designed to limit or prevent initial outbreaks of disease infestations.
- Practical strategies, many already familiar in agriculture, can be combined and optimised to design IDM programmes.
- The goal is preventing disease levels from building up to economically damaging levels.

1. Crop location

- Growing crops in areas best suited to soil, climate and topography provides them with optimal conditions from the start.

- Selection of a suitable site, particularly for perennial crops such as fruit trees, is most important.Stony areas or areas with shallow soils or poor soil texture should be avoided, as these are often associated with a hard pan, which prevents proper root development.
- Soils with poor drainage should also be avoided.

2. Land preparation

- Proper land preparation is important.
- Soil tillage of the field removes hard pans and allows roots to fully penetrate, while a correctly prepared seed bed allows seeds to germinate and grow quickly.
- Improved soil tilth and drainage can reduce nematode levels.
- Tillage can destroy the resting structures and overwintering stages of many diseases.

3. Variety selection

- Undoubtedly, the most attractive form of defense is provided by disease resistance, for as long as it remains effective it provides protection at no cost to the farmer or the community.
- Selection of disease resistance crop varieties has always been a foundation stone of IDM programme.
- Clean, certified seed/root stock is the essential foundation of a healthy crop with a high yield potential.
- No crop management practices are able to compensate for problems arising from poor quality seed or planting material.
- Use clean certified seed and root stock is free of any weed seeds, pests and diseases, for example virus-free tomato seed.
- When establishing an orchard,root stock should be obtained only from a certified nursery.

4. Strategic planting and crop rotation

- Planting similar crops alongside each other should be avoided as it can substantially increase diseases.
- Crop rotations and the previous crops can affect the growth of a crop.
- For example, nematodes can build up with repeated tomato crops in the same field; clover and legumes before another crop puts nitrogen into the soil, reducing the need for applied nitrogen in the following crop; crops such as maize and wheat can reduce the level of Fusarium in the soil.
- Crop rotation helps to minimise the build-up of soil-borne diseases, such as nematodes, weeds (eg Orobanche– Broomrape), diseases (eg Fusarium, and root rots such as Phytopthora and Pythium).

5. Intercropping

- Traditionally, some farmers may sow different crops in alternate rows, or under sow a crop (e. g. maize sorghum) with a legume (e. g. pigeonpea) to manage wilt in pigeonpea.
- Such systems can be labour intensive and difficult to mechanise, but can help reduce disease pressures in individual crops.

6. Soil management

- Ideally an integrated soil fertility management (ISFM) should be adopted.
- ISFM aims to replenish soil nutrient pools, maximize on-farm recycling of nutrients, reduce nutrient losses to the environment and improve the efficiency of external inputs of natural or artificial fertilizer.
- Wrongly timed or excess fertilizer can promote vegetative and dense plant growth which encourages diseases.
- Excess nitrogen fertiliser weakens plants and makes them susceptible to diseases such as mildews and blights.

7. Water management

- Wrongly timed or excess irrigation can promote vegetative plant growth which encourages diseases *viz.*, blight and orobanche in tomatoes, root rot in citrus and faba beans and blight in apple.
- The trunks of citrus trees should not come into contact with irrigation water in order to avoid gummosis.
- Irrigation water must also meet the necessary criteria of hygiene (not obtained from drainage or sewage canals) and salinity, must not contain harmful materials such as heavy metals.

8. Post-harvest sanitation

- Crop residues left in the field can provide shelter for over-wintering diseases such as blights and mildews.
- Crop residues, fallen fruit etc, should be ploughed-in, burnt, or buried.

9. Preserving biodiversity

- Protecting natural habitats near farm area is the best way to conserve biodiversity.
- Careful management of farm land margins, as well as growing trees or hedges, are particularly important because they not only provide habitat, cover and refuge for beneficial insects and other animals but also contribute to the conservation of flora and fauna.

II. Observation

The aim of observation is to determine if, when and what action should be taken to maximize crop production and optimise quality at harvesting. This involves

- Crop monitoring.
- Decision support systems to interpret the data.
- Decision tools, such as "expert systems".
- Remote sensing technologies.

1. Crop monitoring

- Management of any crop requires routine inspections to assess how well plants are growing and what actions need to be taken on cultivations, fertilizer use, disease control, as well as when to harvest.
- Monitoring for diseases is an important part of the need to " walk" through a crop. There is a need to be able to distinguish between disease, non-disease and beneficial species.
- Various tools, diagnostics and forecasting systems are available to assist disease monitoring, minimise the time required, and achieve acceptable accuracy in determining changes in disease infestation.

Basic principles of monitoring/scouting

- Take samples from several areas of the field.
- Select sample sites at random, unless field conditions suggest uneven disease distribution.
- Donot sample in border rows or field edges unless indicated to do so for a particular disease

2. Decision support systems

- Farmers need assistance in interpreting disease monitoring data.
- Simple "expert systems" can be designed and made available to farmers in a range of ways, including simple peg boards or charts, special booklets, radio and television programmes or more advanced aids such as prediction models and computer based systems.
- Development and provision of up-to-date information is a key factor in enabling farmers to implement IDM programmes.

3. Area-wide management

- IDM often requires collaborative decisions within a national or more localized area to provide effective control of diseases.
- Some of these decisions need to be taken centrally by governments in relation to:

- Quarantine regulations and legislation.
- Provision and training of advisory services.
- Strategies for control of highly mobile diseases (e. g. rusts).

Geographical Information Systems (GIS) and remote sensing techniques can also assist in implementation of area-wide management.

III. Intervention

Reducing economically damaging diseases to acceptable levels may involve cultural, physical, biological and chemical control measures individually or in combination. costs, benefits, timing, labor force and equipment as well as economic, environmental and social impacts all have to be taken into consideration.

1. Cultural control

- Serve in promoting the healthy growth of the crop.
- Effective in directly reducing inoculums potential.
- Enhancing the biological activities of antagonists in the soil.
- Cultivation practices such as intercropping, planting date, plant density, crop rotation, roughing, healthy planting material, soil solarization, soil amendments, water management, fertilizer management have been used singly and in combination as tools for disease management.
- For some crops, such control practices may be the only economically viable method available.

2. Mechanical control

- Mechanical methods are the first options to consider when disease reach an unacceptable level.
- They include simple hand picking, hot water and steam treatment, soil solarization and tillage to disrupt breeding.
- The possibility of integrating cultural and physical techniques with the careful use of crop protection products should be explored.
- For example, instead of doing seed treatment entirely with fungicides, solar heat and hot water treatment may be used in conjunction with them.

3. Biological control

- Biological control is nature's own methods of disease control.
- Natural biological processes and material can provide control, with minimal environment impact, and often at low cost.
- The main focus here is on promoting bioagents that control target diseases.
- Biological fungicides derived from naturally occurring microorganism (e.g Trichoderma and Pseudomonas) also fit into this category.

- Research on biological control is yielding new useful products and methods which can be integrated into IDM programmes.
- However, biological products are generally too often unreliable or not efficient enough in the field to be commercially used on their own.
- Biological control also need similar technical expertise as chemical agents in respect to formulation, field application and resistance management.
- Combining biological and chemical control is achieved through selection of the appropriate chemical active ingredient or formulation type, or separating their use over time.
- The most common is Trichoderma, used to control various important diseases like wilt, root rot , collar rot etc.
- The spectrum of activity is narrow compared with most synthetic chemicals, and this is useful in IDM strategies.

4. Chemical control

- Fungicides played an important role in disease control for many decades.
- As component of an IDM ,chemical control are still the most cost –effective way of managing disease, if used judiciously.
- The contact fungicides such as mancozeb, chlorothalonil, copper and sulphur based products continued to have a good share of the market in India because of their lower cost.
- However, systemic fungicides started gradually to replace the older non systemic chemicals with more effectiveness and specificity in disease control.
- Of late, new classes of fungicides were developed with significant impact on disease control. These include tirazoles, strobilurins and activators of systemic acquired resistance.
- The availability of a variety of new products , with narrow and broad specificity, offer important disease control options.The fungicidal application had a better impact when used within an IDM strategy.
- The fungicide industry is focusing in developing effective products with low mammalian toxicity and environmental impact and low residues in food, to meet international health standards and compatibility in IDM programs.
- They must be applied correctly to get the most out of these products.
- Judicious use and superior handling practices limit potential pesticides residue in crops and the environment and help to avoid disease resistance and resurgence.
- Farmers must use advanced equipment and improved application techniques *viz.*, spot spraying, reduced drift nozzles etc. to protect natural habitats for natural and wildlife enemies.

4. Biotechnological interventions

- Biotechnological interventions have substantial potential to contribute to IDM.
- Development of crop varieties resistant to diseases has been the first and most rapidly expanding area of biotechnology for disease control.

8

Principles and Strategy of Plant Disease Management

The techniques used in disease management mainly based on two principles,: *Prevention or prophylaxis* and *cure*The first principle prevention includes *disease management tactics applied before infection* i.e., *the plant is protected from disease.* It includes: avoidance, exclusion, eradication, resistant&protection. Second principle curative action: *functions with any measure applied after the plant is infected*i.e., *the plant is treated for the disease.*It includes *therapy*

Principles of plant disease management

Prophylaxis	Avoidance	Prevent disease by selecting a time of the year or a site where there is no inoculum or where the environment is not favorable for infection
	Exclusion	Prevent the introduction of inoculums
	Eradication	Eliminate, destroy or inactivate the inoculums
	Protection	Prevent infection by means of a toxicant or some other barrier to infection
	Resistance	Utilize cultivars that are resistant to or tolerant of infection
Curative	Therapy	Cure plants that are already infected

1. Avoidance of pathogen : *Avoiding disease by planting at times when or where inoculum is absent or ineffective due to unfavorable environment conditions.*

- Choice of geographic area
- Selection of field
- Choice of time of sowing
- Disease escaping varieties
- Selection of seed and planting stock
- Modification of cultural practices

1. **Exclusion of inoculum:** *Preventing the inoculum from entering or establishing in the field or area where it does not exist.*
    - Seed treatment
    - Inspection and certification

- Quarantine
- Eradication of insect vectors

3. **Eradication of pathogens** : *Reducing, inactivating, eliminating or destroying inoculum at the source, either from a region or from an individual plant in which it is already established.*
    - Biological control of plant pathogen
    - Crop rotation
    - Removal or destruction of diseased plant organs
    - Rouging
    - Eradication of alternate and collateral hosts
    - Sanitation
    - Heat and chemical treatment of disease plants
    - Soil treatments
4. **Resistant:** *Utilize cultivars that are resistant to or tolerant of infection.* Resistant varieties, If available you can manage disease at zero cost
5. **Protection measures**: *Preventing infection by creating a chemical toxic barrier between the plant and the pathogen* is comes under protection measures
    - Chemical treatment
    - Chemical control of insect vectors
    - Modification of environments
6. **Therapy**: *Reducing severity of disease in an infected individual*

- *Chemotherapy:The application of chemicals to an infected or diseased plants to stops the infection.* For instance; heat or chemical treatment of propagating materials *viz.*, corms, bulbs and cuttings to eliminated bacteria, fungi, nematodes or viruses that are established within the plant material.
- *Heat therapy*: Hot water treatment of rice seed at51-53°C for 15 min after dipping for 1 d in cool water for management of white tip disaesce caused by *Aphlenchoides besseyi*
- *Tree surgery*: Use of chaubatia paste after pruning of diseasesd parts in horticultural crops.

While these principles are valid today, in the context of modern concepts of plant disease management, they have some critical shortcomings like

- The principles of plant disease control are stated in absolute terms like *exclude, prevent* and *eliminate* that imply a goal of *zero disease*. Plant disease control in this sense in not practical, and in most cases is note even possible. Indeed, we need not eliminate a disease; we merely need to reduce progress and keep *disease development below an acceptable level*. Instead of plant disease control, we need to think in terms of *plant disease management*.

- These principles donot take consideration the *dynamics of plant disease*, that is the changes in the incidence and severity of disease in time and space. We need some means of assessing *quantitatively* the effects of various control measures, singly and in combination on the progress of disease.
- Finally, these principles of plant disease control tend to emphasize *tactics* without fitting them into an *adequate overall strategy*.
- Does this mean that we should abandon the traditional principles? Of course not; We merely have to fit them into an appropriate overall strategy based on epidemiological principles.

Strategies versus Tactics

The dictionary definitions of the two terms are similar, but generally speaking, *an overall plan for reaching a particular objectives is called strategy*, while the *specific means for implementing a given strategy* are called *tactics*. What is a strategy at one level of focus could be called a tactic at another level of focus.

Strategy of disease management

It is well accepted that complete eradication of a pathogen from the earth of the ecosystem is very difficult and against the law of nature. Therefore, the strategy for disease management should be to reduce *the population of pathogen below permissible level* so they do not cause damage. Keeping this in mind, the strategy of disease management should integrate all known methods taking into account the following factors.

1. Pathogen inhibition
2. Tolerable losses
3. Economical control
4. Long term control
5. Collective approach

1. **Pathogen inhibition:** As complete eradication of a pathogen is not possible, there should be more emphasis on to develop a technology which maintain their population below the damaging level.
2. **Tolerable losses:** means tolerate the level of disease that do not harm economically: For example, in crops raised for seed two per cent disease infection is permissible, whereas in crops raised for consumption the permissible limit is 5 per cent.
3. **Economical control:** The strategy for disease management should be implemented after considering the *cost benefit ratio*. The return per unit of money spent must be sufficiently high.
4. **Long term control:** The strategy of disease management should attempt to utilize methods which have a *long term effect* so as to reduce the expenses and pollution of the environment.

5. **Collective approach:** Disease control cannot be achieved by a single farmer since pathogen can move from field to field. Hence, *collective area wise approach is necessary* for effective control.

Any war cannot be won only on quantity of weapons available. Success only comes from a well planned strategy involving the best use of weapons in a coordinated manner at the right time and with proper methods. Similarly, the war against diseases can be won provided an *integrated approach is employed and all the five basic factors discussed above are taken into account.*

9

Methods of Plant Disease Management

Why Crop Protection

The Food and Agriculture Organization (FAO) estimates that up to 40% of food crops are lost due to plant pests and diseases annually. Such losses not only threaten global food security but also have the potential to limit food access due to unavailability of food, or sharp increases in food prices. But this challenge is also an opportunity to find new ways to help crops better withstand adverse conditions in a farmer's field.

That's why scientists are exploring new ideas that can help farmers with tailored solution to save their crops. Public and private sectors offering a broad range of biological, chemical and digital solutions to help farmers safely and responsibly protect their crops from pests and diseases. Diverse and growing portfolio provides farmers with the modern technologies and a wide range of choices for their crop protection needs. These includes innovations like pesticides, herbicides, microbials and digital tools. They also work collaboratively with farmers to offer tailored solutions – including agronomic recommendations based on the specific needs of their fields, crops, and soil to defend against diseases and pests, improve soil health and help to ensure productive harvests, all while protecting our natural resources. Of late,there has been a sustained efforts to trim down Crop Protection Products (CPP) and instead go back to managing agriculture the way it was done centuries ago. The solution is not in shunning chemical pesticides but in educating farmer about proper use and consistently spending on research to come out with safer and more efficient products. Commenting on the affordability of Crop Protection Products, Dr Dalwai Committee report, on "Doubling Farmers Income" mentions that cost of pesticides is only 0.4% of total cost incurred by the farmers. The share of pesticides in the cost of cultivation was 3 per cent in cotton, 1.9 per cent in paddy, further lower in wheat (0.7%) and sugarcane (0.3%). The methods of plant disease management are

9.1 Physical Management

1. Definition

- *Management of plant diseases using physical means is called physical control.*
- Also called *physical therapy* or *thermotherapy*
- It is mostly *curative* in nature

2. Principles

The principles involved in physical control or thermotherapy is that the pathogens present in seed, soil, or planting material.

- Are inactivated or eliminated at temperatures nonlethal for the host tissues.
- Heat causes inactivation and not immobilization of the pathogen by heat.
- The rate at which the pathogen is inactivated is determined by temperature, the higher the temperature, the faster is the inactivation.

3. Methods

Physical methods are employed for reduction or elimination of primary inoculums that may be present in seed, soil, or planting material are

i. Hot water treatment (HWT)
ii. Hot air treatment (HAT)
iii. Steam and Aerated steam therapy (AST)
iv. Moist hot air treatment
v. Solar heat treatment (SHT)

I. Hot water treatment (HWT)

- Hot water treatment is widely used for the control of seed borne pathogens, especially bacteria and viruses.
- For example.

Control of seed borne pathogens through hot –water treatment

Crop	Disease	Causal Organism	Seed Treatment
Rice	White tip	*Aphlenchoides besseyi*	51-53°C for 15 min after dipping for 1 d in cool water.
Pearl millet	Downy mildew	*Sclerospora graminicola*	55°C for 10 min.
Cauliflower & Cabbage	Black rot	*X. campestris pv. campestris*	50°C for 20 min.

- Main drawback in the hot water treatment is that the seeds may be killed or loose its germinability, if the period of treatment exceeds the specified time.

ii. Hot air treatment (HAT)

- Hot air treatment is less effective than hot water treatment but less injurious to seed and easy to operate.
- It has been used against several diseases of sugarcane and is employed for treating canes which are soft and succulent.
- Hot air treatment at 54°C for 8h, effectively eliminates RSD pathogen without impairing the germination of buds.

- Similarly, grassy shoot disease of sugarcane has also been controlled by hot air at 54^{0}C for 8 h.

iii. Steam and aerated steam therapy (AST)

- The use of aerated steam is more effective than hot air and safer than hot water in controlling seed borne infections.
- The heat capacity of water vapour is about half that of water and 2.5 that of air, hence air temperature and time required may be higher than that of hot water and lower than that of hot air.
- The advantages of this method include easier drying of seeds, low loss in germination, easy temperature control and no damage to seed coat of legumes.
- Sugarcane setts are also exposed to aerated steam at 50^{0}C for 3 hrs to eliminate mosaic virus.

iv. Moist hot air treatment (MHAT)

- This method is effectively used in sugarcane to eliminate grassy shoot disease.
- Initially the setts are exposed to hot air at 54^{0}C for 8 hrs, then exposed to aerated steam at 50 ^{0}C for 1 hr and finally to moist hot air at 54^{0}C for 2 hours.

v. Solar heat treatment (SHT)

- Solar heat treatment is effective in controlling both seed borne and soil borne diseases.
- It has been devised in India to eliminate the pathogen of loose smut of wheat.
- Luthra in 1953 devised a method in India to eliminate the deep seated infection of *ustilago nuda.* The method is popularly known as *solar heat or solar energy treatment.*
- In this method the seeds are soaked in cold water for 4 hours in the forenoon on a bright summer day followed by spreading and drying the seeds in hot sun for four hours in the afternoon. Then, the seeds are again treated with carboxin or carbendazin at 2g/kg and stored.
- This method is highly useful for treating large quantities of the seed lots.

4. Soil Solarization

- Defined as hydrothermal treatment of soil for management of soil borne diseases.
- In this management tactics, the solar energy is preserved with the help of transparent polythene sheet for about 40 days to increase soil temperature (10-15^{0}C) above normal temperature enough to kill the most of the soil borne diseases.

Results of solarization

- Increased soil temperature.
- Improved soil physical and chemical features.
- Control of pests.
- Encouragement of beneficial soil organisms.
- Increased plant growth.
- Fungal diseases such as damping off, root and stem rots, wilt and blights diseases and some nematodes have been successfully managed by soil solarization.

5. Refrigeration

- The low temperature at or slightly above the freezing point checks the growth and activities of all such pathogens that cause a variety of post harvest diseases of vegetables and fruits.
- Therefore most perishable fruits and vegetables should be transported and stored in refrigerated vehicles and stores to manage post harvest diseases.

9.2 Cultural Management

Introduction

At present, the situation is quite different from those early days of disease management. The social climate is demanding reduced dependence on toxic chemicals to solve problems. Such concern have developed as a result of detection of residue in the environment, frequent pesticide accidents, drinking water and food contamination, the growing interest in the food quality, human health and growing organic food market , the decreasing effectiveness of many pesticides as more and more disease become resistant to them .Disease management scientists have responded to this situation by promoting a philosophy of intergraded disease management.

At the outset, IDM approaches emphasized the able used of pesticides. However, problems often arise even when pesticides are use as recommended. Most correctly applied pesticides still misses its target. As of these and other plight associated with pesticides it seems rational to anticipate that we will sooner or later have to restrict their use .

The next approach in the development of IDM was to search for more safe substitutes for pesticides; biological control, biotechnological and digital approaches, etc. Such approaches, even though useful as less invasive curative methods, still avoid confronting the causes of the problem.

A third phase in the development of IDM systems that recognizes diseases not as enemies, but as indicators of problems in the design and management of systems. The ecological knowledge holds most of the keys to suitable environmental designs and methods of management capable of keeping disease loss below unacceptable levels.

The potential range of cultural and bio-ecological controls comes under this approach. The more familiar chemical control are then reserved for emergencies.

Further advances in this approach are dependent on identifying and responding to the barriers to the development and implementation of cultural methods of disease management. Key among these are the lack of appropriate research, training, services, equipment and cultivars. Apart from these, changes in human values and attitudes will also be required; a shift in emphasis from cosmetic to nutritional quality; and from disease elimination to management below thresholds related to our values.

Cultural controls do not offer a panacea for disease prevention and control. This approaches range from the environmentally supportive, knowledge and skill intensive techniques like the optimal design and management of agro ecosystems in time and space to the more heavy handed interventions that can result in soil erosion and environmental degradation.

Cultural control

- Oldest method of disease control.
- Management of disease through agronomical manipulation is called cultural control.
- Preventative in nature.
- It employs practice that make the environment less attractive to diseases and less favorable for their survival, dispersal, growth and reproduction and that promote the natural controls.
- The objective is to achieve reduction in disease losses, either below economic injury levels, or sufficiently to allow natural or biological control to take effect.

Basic principles of cultural practices for disease control

The basic principles of cultural practices for disease control are

- Any potential control method may be considered, providing that it is environmentally, technologically and economically feasible.
- Pesticide usage is minimized by combining with other non-chemical or chemical methods.
- Diseases that are difficult to control or that involve problematic pesticides, e.g. methyl bromide, should be prioritized.
- Economic aspects are taken into consideration.

Advantages

- Ecofriendly and cheaper.
- Only require modifications to normal production practices.
- Specific to a particular disease.

- Self sustaining management.
- Works most of the time.
- Effective and profitable for high acreage of low value crops.
- Dependable, and are usually specific.
- Do not possess some of the detrimental side effects of pesticides.

Disadvantages

- Can sometimes fail in its specificity.
- Slow method of disease management.
- Expensive at startup.
- Needed long term planning for greatest effectiveness.
- More demanding on the farmer's competence.
- Do not always provide complete economic control of diseases.

Cultural controls include:

A. Selection of site

B. Plant design & management

- Crop isolation
- Planting density
- Mixed cropping
- Timing of seeding & planting
- Crop rotations
- Sowing depth
- Fallowing
- Spacing
- Destructions of volunteer plant
- Replacement of alternate hosts
- Management of trap crops

C. Maintenance of site

- Cultivation, tillage
- Plant nutrient management
- Pruning defoliation, thinning & topping
- Irrigation
- Sanitation
- Mulches

- Crop free period and crop free zone
- Creating barriers by non-host or dead hosts
- Soil solarization

D. Production and use of pathogen free planting material

- Proper drying and storage of seeds
- Cleaning of seed
- Adjustment of harvesting time
- Seed production areas
- Inspection of seed production areas

Description of the methods

A. Selection of site

- Disease can be avoided by selecting a planting site that is ideal for the crop and the natural enemies of the disease, but adverse for the disease itself.
- Factors to be considered include the history of the site, its proximity to potential overwintering sites (hedges, field border, woodlots etc.) or sites with abundant natural controls(field border, hedges, woodlots etc), microclimate, climate, topography, elevation, soil conditions, weed species etc.
- When plants are grown in stressed conditions, they tend to emit signals that attract certain diseases.
- One key is to avoid stressing the crop.

B. Planting design and management

1. Crop isolation

- This practice is most suitable for annual crops, particularly when climatic conditions are not ideal.
- Isolation is one way of reducing the probability of attack from the disease.
- Isolation from old crops of the same type and from closely related indigenous host-plants that act as source of diseases is one way of reducing the probability of attack.
- The degree of isolation and location of crops with respects to one another can affect their likelihood of being invaded by diseases.
- Separation of sequentially planted crops in time to disrupt host –plant continuity and prevent easy diseases dispersal may be useful.

2. Crop rotation

- In plant pathology, crop rotation means using plant to manage plant pathogens.
- If a particular crop is grown continuously on the same piece of land, the crop gets disease easily, because pathogens survive due to regular presence of susceptible host.
- Regular crop rotation can control the diseases in the following ways.
  - The physical, chemical and biological effects of different crops cause unfavorable soil environment to the pathogens.
  - The survival ability of pathogen in soil is limited.
  - By changing the crop every year, their population can be reduced by starvation due to lack of host.
  - Better growth of crop plants due to better nutrient availability also helps in avoiding disease.
- For example, Crop rotation helps to minimise the build-up of soil-borne diseases, such as nematodes, weeds (eg Orobanche– broomrape), diseases (eg Fusarium, and root rots such as Phytopthora and Pythium).
- Legumes such as Crotataria and Stylosanthes spp. have also been used to reduce populations of the nematode *Pratylenchus* spp. in soils.
- Similarly, Tagetes spp. (marigolds) inhibit the development of a range of nematode species.
- Many brassica crops produce glucosinolates that break down to produce isothiocyanates which are active against several soil-borne pathogens.

3. Fallowing

- Fallowing, is the mode of preparing land, by ploughing it a considerable time before it is ploughed for seed.
- It is normally adopted in plant disease management for killing pathogens persisting in soil or in crop residues.
- For fallowing the field should remain weed free.
- Though fallowing is an alternative method for reducing pathogen population it is often resorted to because of the economic consideration.
- Fallowing is of three types: (a) dry fallowing, (b) wet fallowing and (c) flood fallowing.

a. Wet fallowing

- In wet fallowing frequent irrigation is given during the fallow period. It is usually practiced for some weeks.
- The main aim is to make the pathogen germinate in the soil which later dies due to lack of host plant.

- Wet fallowing reduced the pathogen population especially of sclerotia which retains viability in dry conditions for several years.
- It is also partly successful in reducing the population of *Pythium* and *Alternaria* .

b. Dry fallowing

- Dry fallowing is generally used where other methods of dis-infestation of soil pathogens are not economical.
- In this method the field is kept as such for a period of one season to kill the pathogen by starvation.

c. Flood fallowing

- In flood fallowing the land is kept submerged and the pathogens die due to lack of oxygen.
- Rotting of plant debris also releases materials toxic to pathogens.

4. Mixed cropping

Mixed cropping is growing of two or more crops simultaneously on the same piece of land. It reduces the economic loss from diseases. The reduction in disease incidence in a mixed crop can be attributed to following causes.

- Due to reduced number of host plants there is sufficient spacing between them and chances of contact between foliage or roots of diseased and healthy plants are greatly reduced.
- The roots of non host plants may act as a physical barrier obstructing the movement of pathogen in soil. They may also release toxic substances in their root exudates which suppress the growth of pathogens attacking the main crop. HCN in root exudates of sorghum is toxic to *F udum* attacking pigeon pea in the mixture.
- Due to reduced number of host pants in a mixed crop the susceptible area for an air borne foliar pathogen is decreased. Therefore, there is less primary infection and less production of secondary inoculums for spread of the disease. This slow down the rate of disease control.
- By proper selection of crops for the mixture, soil environment can also be changed to one that is not favorable for the pathogen. Control of root rot of cotton by growing cotton with moth is an example.
- The soil borne pathogens are not uniformly distributed in the field soil. Generally they are randomly present as dormant structures. Activation of these dormant structures is often dependent on contact with host roots. The chances of which are highly reduced in mixed crop due to spacing between plants.

5. Adjustment of sowing dates

- The sowing time is adjusted in such a way that it reduces the infection period of a pathogen to meet the susceptible stage of the host plant to the minimum.
- It can be achieved by changing the date of sowing so that the susceptible stage of plant growth does not coincide with the environments highly favorable for the pathogen.
- Bunt of winter wheat can be controlled by either planting before mid September or after mid October.
- Early planting of potatoes enables the crop to reach tuberization stage before the insect *viz.* aphid, reaches it peak in the months of January.
- But this sowing time adjustment also has some disadvantages. For example, late sown pea can reduce the extent of early root rot and wilt, but during pod formation stage in late sown pea, powdery mildew and rust will affect the crop.
- Therefore the farmer has to select the planting date according to the importance of a particular disease in his locality.

6. Sowing depth

- Sowing depth can also be adjusted with due regard for soil type and moisture to shorten the period of emergence and to reduce the incidence of damping off disease in many crops.
- In heavy soil, seed should be placed shallow as compared to light soils.
- Similarly, in dry soil the seed should be placed deeper in the moist zone, while if water is available irrigate the field before sowing of the a few centimeters and then sow the seeds.
- Depth of sowing is usually determined by seed size and the moisture status of the soil.
- Deeper sowing may promote germination but it also lengthens the (usually) susceptible pre-emergence seedling phase.
- Smuts and seedling diseases caused by *Fusarium* spp. and *Rhizoctonia* spp. are more serious if seeds are planted deeply.
- Similarly potato seed pieces are more readily attacked by Rhizoctonia if planted too deeply.

7. Spacing

- Of late, the production technology emphasizes on high plant population for getting high yields.
- But it facilitates luxuriant plant growth, which can cause disease.
- Luxuriant vegetative growth due to high fertilizer dose, humidity and solar radiation combined with lack of aeration and light to plants, invites pathogen and favors their rapid growth.

- Damping off ,late blight of potato and mildew of grape vines are some of the diseases which spread fast in close spaced plantings.
- But there are also examples where dense sowing help in disease reduction.
- For example, virus of leaf curl disease of tomato transmitted by white fly is less in crowded planting than in wide spaced planting.
- The same is true for cucumber mosaic and groundnut rosette transmitted aphids. Incidence of fungal disease of brown rot of soybean and wilt in cotton is reduced in close sown crop.

8. Destruction of volunteer plants

- Volunteer plants can help to perpetuate a disease problem by furnishing a food source to long life cycled diseases of preceding crops.
- They are very attractive to many diseases and serve as the focal point for future infestations.
- It is therefore desirable to destroy volunteer plants to assist in the disease control.

9. Management of alternate hosts

- Diseases reproduce on alternate and alternative hosts and then attack the main crops.
- Therefore it is desirable to destroy alternated hosts like barberry for management of black stem rust or other weeds on barren land to assist in the control of insects like aphids, leafhoppers etc.

10. Management of trap and decay crops

- Trap and decoy crops are susceptible plants that are grown on land known to contain various pathogens.
- The pathogens infect the crop which must be destroyed before the life cycles of the pathogens are complete.
- Trap crops can be grown simultaneously with more valuable crops.
- The efficiency of trap crops in reducing the spread of pathogens depends on the plant, growth habit differences including height differentials and position relative to the'protected' crop.
- Decoy crops stimulate the hatching of nematode eggs or the germination of resting structures or seeds of other pathogens, but the pathogens are unable to establish a compatible relationship with the decoy crop host and eventually die.
- As a result, the level of inoculum of the pathogen declines. For example, ryegrass reduces the incidence of clubroot of crucifers (*Plasmodiophora brassicae*) in infested soil while the poisonous weed thorn apple (*Dahra stramonium*) reduces the incidence of powdery scab of potatoes (*Spongospora subterranea*).

- Ideally, a decoy crop would be of economic value and may be included in a normal crop rotation..

11. Strip farming

- This practice separates areas of one crop with intervening strips of another crop or fallow.
- The rationale for adopting strip farming practices is that crops in adjacent strips rarely share common pathogens.
- The rates of spread of more specialized parasites are also restricted because of the discontinuous distribution of suitable hosts.
- The major problems associated with strip farming are increased costs of production relative to monocultures, selection of crops for adjacent strips which have few common parasites and weed control between the strips.
- Strip farming has an additional role in reducing soil erosion.

C. Maintenance of site

1. Tillage

This approach can help in the control of soil inhabiting diseases by:

- Bringing resting structures, spores, conidia ,sclerotia etc onto the soil surface, thereby exposing them to desiccation and predation, freezing and thawing.
- Damaging the pathogens in its soil inhabiting phase.
- Destroying crop residues, which might harbour diseases that could invade new crops.
- Burying residues so deep that emergence from resting structure is made impossible.

2. Plant nutrient management

- Ideally an integrated soil fertility management (ISFM) should be adopted.
- ISFM aims to replenish soil nutrient pools, maximize on-farm recycling of nutrients, reduce nutrient losses to the environment and improve the efficiency of external inputs of natural or artificial fertilizer.
- Wrongly timed or excess fertiliser can promote vegetative and dense plant growth which encourages pests such as aphids and whitefly.
- Excess nitrogen fertilizer weakens plants and makes them susceptible to pests such as aphids and whitefly, and diseases such as mildews and blights.

3. Timing of tillage and fertilization operations

- This may affect diseases favorably or unfavorably.
- Efforts should be made to avoid damage and stress to plants, and also over

fertilization, thereby avoiding making the crop particularly attractive and susceptible to diseases.

4. Irrigation

- Wrongly timed or excess irrigation can promote vegetative plant growth which encourages pests and diseases such as aphids and whitefly in cotton, blight and orobanche in tomatoes, root rot in citrus and faba beans, and spider mite, aphids and blight in apple.
- The trunks of citrus trees should not come into contact with irrigation water in order to avoid gummosis.
- As examples, wet soil favours club root of crucifers, silver scurf of potatoes and Cercosporella on wheat, while dry soil increases severity of white mold of onion, common scab of potato and Fusarium diseases of cereals.
- Irrigation water must also meet the necessary criteria of hygiene (not obtained from drainage or sewage canals) and salinity, must not contain harmful materials such as heavy metals.

5. Soil solarization

- Soil solarization is non chemical management procedure adopted by farmers in several parts of the country.
- It is an advanced field technology for the management of soil borne pathogens, weeds and improves soil suppressiveness and fertility.
- Soil solarization is based on the trapping solar irradiation by tightly covering the soil, usually with transparent polythene sheets.
- This results in increase in temperature up to the point (10-15°C above normal) where most pathogens are vulnerable to heat effects.
- Major fungal diseases managed successfully include damping off, root rots, stem rots, fruit rots, major parasitic fungi and diseases managed successfully include damping off, wilt , blight, root rots, stem rots, fruit rots.
- Major nematode successfully managed are *Ditylenchus dipsaci, Globodera rostochiensis, Heterodera,* and *Meloidogyne* etc.
- Bacterial canker of tomato successfully controlled by solarization for 1-2 months.

6. Pruning, defoliation and topping

- Destruction and removal of dead, diseased or infested parts during the dormant phase can greatly reduce overwintering stages of pathogens and thus their spread the next year. e.g., scale and fire blight infested terminals.

7. Sanitation

- Field and plant sanitation is a main part of disease control through cultural practices.
- This step is essential even if disease or pathogen free seed or propagating material has been used and other recommended cultural practices have been followed.
- The inoculums present on few plants in the field may nullify in soil or on the plant and in due course of time may be sufficient to nullify the effect of other cultural practices.
- Therefore, plants bearing such pathogens or plant debris introducing the inoculums in the soil should be removed as early as feasible.
- For instance, wilt disease pathogen of banana remains in dead roots, rhizomes and upper portions of the plant.
- When these plant remains are removed there is rapid decline in the population of the pathogen in the soil.
- Similarly, the wilt of cotton and arhar and root rot of bean are also reduced to some extent by removal of diseased plant debris.

a. Removal of crop debris

- The plant stubbles and roots, left in the field form most of the crop debris.
- The infected crop debris not only harbours pathogen but also provides media for their growth.
- The fungus of downy mildew of pea, jowar, bajara and maize, powdery mildew of pea and cereals are some of the diseases which remain in crop debris after harvesting the diseases crop.
- Destruction of crop debris by burning immediately after harvest reduces the amount of innoculum surviving through debris.
- Deep ploughing during hot summer (after rabi crop) burries the debris to such depth where pathogen is destroyed easily.
- Turning of soil also exposes the pathogen present in the deeper zone, to hot temperature during day time and kills them.
- Letting the field fallow for some time also serves this purpose as pathogen die to starvation.

b. Elimination of volunteer/alternate host plants

- Crop plants remaining from previous seasons and volunteer host plants that establish in fallowed land or around cropping areas when climatic conditions are suitable during intercrop periods may provide sources of inoculum for succeeding crops.

- Unwanted crop plants should be destroyed by either cultivation or the application of herbicides.
- Weeds or wild plants may act as alternative hosts of plant parasites allowing the pathogen to survive between seasons and providing a source of inoculum in the new growing season. For example, grasses such as *Hordeum leportnum* are hosts of the wheat take-all fungus *Gaeumannomyces graminis.*
- Some rusts cannot complete their life cycles in the absence of alternate hosts, One important macrocyclic cereal rusts, *Puccinia graminis* require alternate hosts (*Berberis* spp.) to complete their life cycles.
- So,there has been a concerted effort to eradicate *Berberi.* spp to manage the disease

c. Removing diseased plants or plant parts

- Removing diseased plants or plant parts to eliminate sources of inoculum is carried out routinely in many nurseries, green houses and high-value crops.
- Diseased parts of larger plants such as tree crops are often removed by pruning. Infected branches are removed in cases of fireblight of pome fruit, apple canker, powdery mildew of apples and silver leaf of plums .
- Mummified fruit as well as diseased twigs should be removed from pome and stone fruits to reduce the inoculum of Sclerotinia spp.
- Subsequent sanitation measures usually involve burning pruned material and treating cut surfaces with suitable fungicides.
- Pruning inevitably influences the microclimate within the tree canopy indirectly affecting any subsequent disease development.

d. Crop free period and crop free zone

- The pathogen attacking crops of secondary importance and having a narrow host range can be controlled by maintaining a crop free period of definite duration.
- When the growers in an area agree not to grow the crops susceptible to the pathogen for a definite period, depending on longevity of the pathogen without its host , the pathogen is automatically starved out.
- Similarly, when the host crop is not grown in a zone surrounding the infested area, spread of the disease is checked.
- On this basis , for control of bunchy top of banana, a crop free belt around the area affected by the disease checks it spread provided disease planting material is also quarantined and insect vectors are unable to cross crop free zone.
- This method is effective for those diseases which are not seed borne and either there is no insect vector or if insect vectors spread then their flight range is limited.

e. Creating barriers by non-host or dead hosts

- The spread of majority of diseases from one plant to another in the same field depends on the proximity of healthy roots to infected roots.
- Growing of other crop in between as in mixed cropping creates barrier by the presence of roots of non-host crops in between.
- One of the control measure for bacterial wilt of banana and spreading decline of citrus is to destroy the healthy plants around the diseased plants.
- This checks the movement of pathogen from diseased to healthy plants that are left in the field.

f. Weed management

- Weeds are the alternate host of many pathogens.
- They carry over the pathogen from one season to another and also provide a base from which pathogen is multiplied.
- For instance, powdery mildew of cucurbits persists on wild cucurbit plant during winter season.
- Kans grass is an alternate host of sugarcane smut and downy mildew of sugarcane.

C. Production and use of pathogen free planting material

- Many plant pathogens like bacteria, virus, fungi and nematodes are transmitted by diseased seed or other vegetative propagating parts.
- For successful disease control this source of primary inoculums must be destroyed.
- The following methods are followed to produce and use pathogen free seed material.

1. Proper drying and storage of seeds

- If the seeds are not dried properly before storage they loose their germination capacity and also harbor several types of plant pathogen in it.
- The fungus, causing downy mildew of maize is found to be present in the seed when it is fresh.
- When the seed is thoroughly dried the fungus present in it dies. Prolonged storage of seed also helps in eliminating several pathogens. *Fusarium solani* f. sp. *cucurbitae*, infecting cucurbits, is eliminated if the seeds are stored for 2 years before sowing.
- Proper conditions of storage must be maintained to avoid any harm to the seed.

2. Cleaning of seed

- In many cases the pathogen is present in plant parts mixed with the seed. When such seed are used pathogen easily gets into the field.

- Proper cleaning of seeds before sowing is essential.
- Common examples of diseases disseminated in this manner are ergot and smut of pearl millet, ear cockle of wheat, white rust of crucifers, ascochyta blight of chickpea, etc.

3. Adjustment of harvesting time

- Disease incidence can be minimized by reducing spread of inoculums through adjustment of harvesting time and practice.
- For example, potatoes harvested when the tops are still green may easily get contaminated by late blight fungus present on the leaves.
- One of the practices to avoid tuber contamination or infection is to first remove the green tops and let them dry in the soil for 15 days before digging the tubers.
- When digging of tubers is prolonged the late blight fungus are killed and the produce becomes disease free.

4. Seed production areas

- Seed should be produced in areas where the pathogens of major concerns are unable to establish or maintain themselves at critical levels during periods of seed development.
- Area with low relative humidity and low rainfall are favorable for production of high quality seeds.
- Crop infected with diseases like bacterial blight of legumes, ascochyta blight of chickpea and anthracnose of cucurbits, etc. should be grown in dry areas with the help of irrigation.

5. Inspection of seed production areas

- Periodical inspection of crops raised for seed production is an important procedure in the production of clean and healthy seeds.
- Destruction of diseased plants/organs at the time of inspection helps in reducing inoculums in the field and thus, the percentage of healthy seeds in the produce is increased.
- If disease incidence is high, the entire crop may be rejected for seed.

Implementation of cultural controls

The following initiatives will need to be taken for the cultural control to achieve their potential.

- Government must give funding support for the establishment of research related to use of cultural method of disease management .
- Priorities should be given, with emphasis on long term on farm participatory research and multidisciplinary team research.

- Research in this area should be done both in house and through the awarding of grants to researchers.
- Legislation is required to make sure that users are capable in the use of safe alternatives, including the relevant cultural controls.
- Legislation to cooperate in application of certain cultural management programs like destruction of alternate host of certain diseases, pruning of diseased plant parts, rouging etc.
- Governments will need to establish a clear policy on sustainable agriculture and essentially have to identify appropriate strategy for the management of crop diseases.
- Support should be provided to Agriculture Universities for the establishment of courses in cultural control and for the preparation of appropriate teaching materials and demonstration plots.
- An intensive and creative public education campaign should be mounted to get these message across.

9.3 Host Plant Resistance

Problems in developing disease management systems

- Development of disease management systems in part determined by economic pressures.
- Resistance and tolerance neglected , as in fruit crops, where inputs and returns per hectare high.
- Need of chemical treatment increased, when qualities of appearance and taste became higher valued by the consumers.
- More demanding the consumer with respect to appearance, the more treatment were needed; in some areas, a crop of apples was economically produced with some thirty treatments per year.
- When more specific and more effective chemicals came on the market, the fungi developed tolerant strains.

For the agricultural annual crops, often with a low cash flow per ha, resistance breeding is the main solution. Three periods can be distinguished tentatively;

1. Pre-mendelian period
2. R-gene period
3. Recent period

1. Pre-mendelian period

The pre-mendelian period may be characterized by

- Low nitrogen levels and mixed cropping.
- Use of landrace cultivars with a fair degree of intrasepcific diversity.

- Subconcious selection toward polygenic resistance.
- Example; maize-rust and potato –late blight pathosystem

2. R-gene period

The R gene period may be characterized by

- Period last from about 1920 to 1970.
- Application of Mendel's laws to plant breeding.
- Selection for monogenic resistance.
- Medium nitrogen level.
- Polygenic resistance at the medium nitrogen level seemed to be less satisfactory than at the low level, induced the change.
- In some pathosystem, plant breeders obtained long term protection against disease by means of monogenic resistance.
- Success; wheat-stem rust pathosystem, with successes in North America.
- Failure: wheat –stripe rust in Europe, rice –blast pathosystem in Japan & Latin America and in the potato –late blight pathosystem.

3. Recent period

- More research effort is spent on partial resistance.
- Success are very few but evident.
- High nitrogen level are a drawback.
- Example: in the potato-late blight pathosystem, plant breeders obtained a high degree of horizontal resistance. After severe epidemic of tropical maize rust (*P. polysora*) on maize in Africa, cultivated maize rapidly developed partial resistance, so that the rust situation came under control again without intervention of any plant breeder.
- Experiment with new systems of gene management have been initiated.

Strengthening the plant immune system

Drawing parallel again with human medical treatment, Ayurved deals with not the symptom but the root cause to make one stronger and deal with the problem through stronger immune response.If we apply the same analogy to crops,we can make plants stronger to develop greater resistance to such attacks through immune response system. This is possible through genetically superior seed developed through natural selection or induced hybridization, as well as by providing right quantum of nutrients to the plant to develop stronger inherent capabilities to fight the disease. This is like the well-fed human who has stronger capabilities to resist attack from different viruses versus the human who is nutrient deficit. Like humans, plants need the right fertilizers and nutrients during its entire period of growth to grow strong.

Definition of Resistance

- Resistance is the ability of a plant to withstand, oppose, lessen, or overcome the attack of a pathogen or
- The inherent ability of an organism (i.e., the crop plant) to resist or withstand the pathogen is called resistance.

Plant resistance to a pathogen results from the expression by the plant of resistance linked characters that obstruct with one or more aspects of the pathogen interaction with the plant. In IDM tactics, host plant resistance entails the intentional use of resistant crop varieties alone or in combination with other tactics, to reduce the impact of disease on crop yield or quality.The traditional approach to the development and use of resistant varieties in IDM involves four steps;

- **Screening** : Evaluation of crop germplasm for identification of resistant varieties.
- **Categorization**: Assignment of categories for resistance, moderately resistance and tolerance.
- **Breeding**:Transfer of candidate genes responsible for resistance into agronomic ally acceptable backgrounds.
- **Implementation**:Integration of resistant varieties into IDM programmes.

Classification of Resistance

Each plant species is affected by hundreds of kinds of pathogen. Frequently a single plant is attacked by hundreds of individuals of a pathogen. Yet, those plants survive which are resistant, adapting a number of mechanisms classified variously.

1. Based on type of host response

a. Immune

- Immunity is exempt from infection or hundred per cent freedom from disease.
- No symptom develop. For instance, potato is resistance to karnal bunt.

b. Resistance

- Resistance characterizes those situations in which some degree of host pathogen interaction is evoked.
- Therefore, resistance is partial, that is ,always some symptoms appear contrary to immunity, where no symptoms appear.

c. Tolerance

- Tolerance is defined as the inherent or acquired capacity of the host to endure disease.
- Tolerance means disease tolerance where yield losses are minimum even in the presence of disease.

- Therefore, tolerance is the capacity of the host genotype to compensate yield losses even when diseases.

2. Based on ecological resistance or pseudo resistance

Apparent resistance resulting from transitory characters in potentially susceptible host plants due to environmental conditions.

Pseudo resistance may be classified into 3 categories

a. Host evasion

- Host may pass through the most susceptible stage quickly or at a time when insects or pathogens are less or evade injury by early maturing.
- This pertains to the whole population of host plant.

b. Induced resistance

- Increase in resistance temporarily as a result of some changed conditions of plants or environment such as change in the amount of water or nutrient status of soil.

c. Escape

- Absence of infestation or injury to host plant due to transitory process like incomplete infestation.
- This pertains to few individuals of host.
- Example; early maturing or short duration variety may escape serious disease attack (wheat rust and potato late blight). Rapid germination of seed and growth of seedling may escape attack by damping off pathogens.. Perceptive growth stage of host may not coincide with conducive condition for disease development(*Botrytis* and *Alternaria* are more severe on old senescing plants)

3. Based on epidemiological terms (number of races controlled)

a. Vertical resistance (VR)

When a plant variety is more resistant to a few races of pathogen than to others, the resistance is called 'vertical' or 'perpendicular' resistane. This types of resistance is called by various names as per reasons given below:

- **Oligogenic resistance:** The resistance is governed by one or few genes.
- **Monogenic resistance:** When the resistance is controlled by single gene.
- **Specific resistance:** When resistance controls only one race of a pathogen.
- **Qualitative resistance:** Because its resistance is simple.
- **Major gene resistance:** Each gene involved in the resistance has distinct effect.
- **Non-uniform resistance:** The host with vertical resistance controls only one race, therefore, it is also known as non uniform resistance.

Vertical resistance is most effective when

1. It is directed against pathogens that do not reproduce and spread rapidly such as Fusarium, or pathogens that donot mature very frequently, such as *Puccinia graminis*.
2. It consists of strong genes that confer complete and long term protection to the pathogen which carries it.
3. It is incorporated in annual crops that are easy to breed, such as small grains.
4. The host population does not consist of a single genetically uniform variety grown over large area.
5. It is recommended for intensive agriculture.
6. Merit lies in its easy handling by breeders.

Vertical resistance becomes short lived if one or more of these and various other conditions are not met. It breakdown as a result of appearance of new pathogen races that can bypass or overcome it.

b. Horizontal resistance (HR)

The resistance of host to all the races of a pathogen is called horizontal resistance. This types of resistance is called by different names as per reasons given below:

- **Polygenic resistance**: When the resistance is controlled by number of genes.
- **General resistance** : The host plant provides protection from all the prevailing races of a pathogen.
- **Quantitative resistance**. Because its resistance is complex.
- **Minor gene resistance**. : Each gene involved in the resistance has small effect which is not visible.
- **Non-specific resistance**: The host resistance is not for a specific race of a pathogen, The resistance is similar to all the races of a pathogen therefore, it is also known as uniform resistance.

Characteristics of HR

- Confer incomplete but more durable protection.
- As most VR, it does not break down as quickly and suddenly.
- Recommended for sustainable agriculture.
- Varieties with HR stay resistant for much longer than do varieties with VR, However, the level of resistance in plant with HR is much lower than in plants with VR.
- HR is universally present in domesticated and wild plants and operates against all races of a pathogen including the most pathogenic ones.
- It involves many host physiological processes that act as mechanisms of defense and that are beyond the limits of its variability.

Mechanism of resistance

The various mechanisms of disease resistance are as follows

1. Mechanical

- Mechanical or structural resistances are due to external or internal peculiarities of the host plant.
- The first line of defense is the surface. Thick hairs, cuticle, wax and hairs on plant parts and foliage check the germination and entry of pathogen in the host tissue.
- The epidermal cells of rice varieties resistant to blast are lignified.
- Formation of cork layer beyond the infection point of *R solani* in potato, or abscission layer around diseased spot in peach against *Xanthomonas pruni* are the few examples to further check the spread of pathogen.

2. Hypersensitivity

- In the large number of cases, immune reaction is due to he hypersensitive reaction of the host.
- The mechanism is found in case of biotrophic organisms or obligate parasites. Immediately after infection, several host cells surrounding the point of infection die.
- This leads to death of the pathogen or at least prevents its spore production.

3. Nutritional

- The reduction in growth and in spore production is generally supposed to be due to an unfavorable physiological conditions within the host.
- Most likely, a resistant host does not fulfill the nutritional requirements of the pathogen and thereby limits its growth and reproduction.

Source of resistance

There are four important sources of disease resistance. These are

1. Cultivated varieties
2. Germplasm collections
3. Wild species
4. Induced mutations

1. Cultivated varieties

- Cultivated varieties are the best sources of disease resistance, because they possess good agronomic characters besides disease resistance.
- Resistance to disease may be found in cultivated varieties of some crops.For example, cotton variety MCU 5 VT tolerant to Verticillium wilt was isolated

from the commercial variety MCU5 of *Gossypium hirsutum.*Some commercial varieties of Asiatic cotton *(G. arboretum)* are good sources of resistance to *Fusarium* wilt.

2. Germplasm collections

- Germplasm collections are the potential sources of disease resistance in all the cultivated crops.
- In cotton, several germplasm lines resistant to bacterial blight and Fusarium wilt have been identified based on screening of large number of germplasm in India.

3. Wild species

- Related wild species are also potential sources of disease resistance.
- Wild species of crops like wheat, barley, potato , tomato, tobacco,cotton etc are good source of resistance to various diseases like leaf rust, yellow rust, powdery mildew, late blight, leaf roll virus, Fusarium wilt, mosaic, TMV, wild fire, bacterial blight etc.Many disease resistance genes have been transferred from wild species to cultivated species in these crops.
- However, utilization of wild sources poses many problems such as cross compatibility, hybrid inviability, hybrid sterility and linkages of several undesirable traits with desirable results.
- Therefore, wild related species are only used as a source of resistance when the desired resistance is not found within the cultivated species.

4. Mutations

- Both spontaneous and induced mutations are good sources of diseae resistance.
- Disease resistance has been achieved in several crops through the use of induced mutations.
- Examples, resistance to Victoria blight and crown rust in oats, to stripe rust in wheat, to mildew in barley, to flax rust in flax etc

Breeding Methods

Breeding methods for disease resistance are the same as for other agronomic characters. The choice of methods depends on source of resistance and mode of pollination of the crop species. Following breeding methods are used for breeding of disease resistance

1. Introduction
2. Selection
3. Hybridization
4. Mutation

1. Introduction

- Introduction is easy and rapid method of developing disease resistant variety.
- Resistant variety may be introduced and after testing, if found suitable, can be released in the disease prone area.
- Grape crop in France was completely destroyed by the attack of *Phylloxera vertifolia* in 1860.
- Introduction of resistant root stocks to this disease from USA saved the grape crop from extinction in France.

2. Selection

- When the source of resistance is a cultivated variety, mass selection and pure lines selection in self pollinated crops, mass selection and progeny selections in cross pollinated crops , and clonal selection in the vegetatively propagated crops will be ideal for isolating disease resistant plants.
- The resistant plants may be multiplied, screened for disease resistance and released as a variety.

3. Hybridization

- Hybridization is used when resistant genes are vailable either in the germplasm or in wild speices of crop plants.
- After hybridization, the hybrid material is handled either by pedigree method or by backcross method.
- The pedigree method is used when the resistance is governed by polygenes and the resistant variety is an adapted one which also contributes some desirable agronomic traits.
- The backcross method is used when the resistant plant is unadapted type or the resistant gene is to be transferred from wild species.
- It is more commonly used when the resistance is governed by oligogenes.

4. Mutation

- Induced mutations are also used for disease resistance.
- Many disease resistance varieties have been developed in various crop through induced mutations.

Vicious Breeding Cycle or Boom and Bust Cycle

The trend in resistance breeding program has been towards increased application of vertical resistance. It can be reasoned that when breeding programs aim at the rapid incorporation of vertical resistance genes, horizontal resistance is diminished. Vanderplank (1963) termed this vertifolia effect . There is evidence that the Vertifolia effect occurred in many pathogsystems among which are the following

Crop	Pathogens	Region
Potato	*Phytophthora infestans*	Many areas
Wheat	*Puccinia graminis*	East Africa
Rice	*Pyricularia oryzae*	Japan, Latin America

Loss of horizontal resistance makes cultivars more vulnerable to new physiologic races. Within a few years the frequency of genes for virulence in the pathogen population compatible to the host's new resistance genes increases. When conditions become favourable the pathogen population builds up and destroys the crop , as an epidemic on a cultivar with little residual resistance will have a high r value. The R gene itself has not changed, but it has lost its economic value.

Agriculture react immediately by introducing another variety with another R gene in all probability again with little residual resistance, whose protection will be overcome by another compatible virugene, and so on. The pathosystem enters a vicious cycle, the boom and bust cycle, to the harm of both farmers and plant breeders. The economic life of a variety is reduced to some three or four years, too short for the farmer to optimize his cropping regimen or for the breeder to gain a decent profit. The boom and bust cycle is best known from pathosystems involving small grains and biotrophic pathogens, for which there were no alternative control methods available until recently. In a milder form this vicious cycle is also known from a number of horticultural pathosystems including some of beans, tomatoes and lettuce.

Escaping from the vicious breeding cycle is not easy. The following possibilities of R-gene management are available:

1. Pyramiding of vertical genes
2. Regional deployment of vertical genes
3. Rotation of vertical gnenes
4. Cultivar mixtures and multiline varieties

1. Pyramiding of vertical genes

- Pyramiding of vertical genes is the accumulation of many vertical genes in one variety.
- It can be successful for two reasons. If n new R-genes are introduced simultaneously, instead of one after the other, the chances that a new and compatible physiologic race will appear decreases to zero. Furthermore, some host species seem to acquire a broader, more horizontal type of resistance when more R –genes accumulate.

2. Regional deployment of vertical genes

- It is the distribution of R-genes by mutual agreement among plant breeders, so that every cropping region has allocated some R-genes that will not be used in other regions.

- Epidemics resulting from inoculums transported by long distance dispersal from another region are avoided in this way.
- This system is operational in the oats-crown rust pathosystem of North America.

3. Rotation of vertical genes

- Rotation of vertical genes may be effective when the fitness of a virugene in the absence of its compatible R-gene is low and r is low.
- For most diseases, it seems to be risky.

4. Multiline varieties

- Intraspecific within field diversity is obtained by producing multiline varieties.
- Success have been achieved in wheat- *Puccinia striiformis*, oats-*Puccinina coronate* and barley- *Erysiphe graminins* .
- The risk taken with this type of diversity is a possible response of the pathogen by pyramiding virugenes so that a superrace is generated.

Resistance as a component of IDM

In integrated disease management philosophy, it is accepted the no single method of disease management, howsoever effective, should be used alone, in long term interest. In IDM diverse options of management are integrated to develop a package which may be location specific. The host resistance, to one or more major diseases, becomes the major focal point around which the IDM strategy is develop. For instance, in potato and wheat, IDM has to start with selection of varieties resistant to late blight and wheat rust, respectively. The minor problems of these crops can be managed by other means of disease management. This is the first stage of integration of host resistance in IDM. The next stage logical approach is the judicious use of fungicides to bring down the initial level of inoculums from which disease starts . This prophylactic spray of fungicide will reduce the initial disease severity and slow down its progress. By adopting this we can take a lot of pressure from host resistance, which will perform efficiently and for longer period. Fry (1983) made significant contribution in management of late blight of potato by integrating host resistance with fungicide application, which work in synergistic manner. Two important points emerged:

- Fungicide requirement of resistant cultivars is significantly reduced (avoiding unnecessary pesticide use).
- Host cultivars not fully resistant can perform reasonably well, if initial fungicide protection is provided.

The generation of scientific information on behavior of host, pathogen, environment and their interaction has enriched our knowledge. With logical thinking this knowledge should be put to use. The consideration is for a long term planning for disease management where host resistance is effectively and economically utilized, as a component of IDM strategy , along with other supporting component.

Resistant variety is nucleus of IDM programmes

- Resistance varieties are the easiest, safest, least expensive and most effective method of disease control in crops.
- Cultivation of resistant varieties eliminates losses from disease and also eliminates expenses for sprays .
- Use of resistant varieties provides a means of managing diseases like vascular pathogens, viruses and root rots that are economically impractical to control.
- It is always preferable to use varieties having both vertical and horizontal resistance,
- Varieties with VR need to be replaced periodically, for instance, after every 3,5or 10 years.
- Genetic engineering technology will allow quick transfer of individual genes or combination of genes for resistance into susceptible crop varieties and thereby reducing the time required to develop a new resistant varieties .
- Even after a resistant variety is released, measure can be taken to prolong its resistance.IDM reduces the exposure of the variety to large pathogen populations is likely to increase its useful life span.
- HPR will not only cause a major reduction in pesticide use and slowdown the rate of development of resistance to pesticides in pathogen populations, but also lead to increased activity of beneficial organisms and reduction in pesticide residues in food and food products.

Tolerant/resistant varieties of major crops

Crop	Name of disease	Resistant/Tolerant varieties
Rice	Blast	Rasi, Vikas, Krishna Hamsa, Tulasi, IR 64, Aditya, Swarnadhan, Himalaya 1, Himalaya 2, Himalaya 2216, Pant dhan 10, HKR 228 and PNR 519
	BLB	Ajaya, IR 36, IR 64, Swarna, Bhumbleshwari, PR 111, PR 113, PR 114, PR 115, PR 116, PR 118, Rajendra Basmati, Pant dhan 11, Govind, Radha, Kamini, Pant dhan 10, Jayshree, Kanchan and improved sambhamasouri.
	Sheath blight	PR 108, Bhudeb Dinesh, Jogan, Mandira, Nalini, Neeraj and Sabita
	RTD	Vikramarya, Nidhi, Amulya, Dinesh, Lakshmi and Nalini
Wheat	Rust	HS 420, HS 277, HS 295, HPW251, VL 892 CPAN 3004, WH 542, HD 2687, PBW 550; WH 896, WH 1105, HD 2964, 8804 HP 1102, UP 262, HUW 206, HP 1102;K 8804 WH 147; GW 190, H 1977GW273, GW322, DL 803-3, Lok 1 HD 2501, MACS 2496, DWR 162, HW 971, HW 2022

Crop	Name of disease	Resistant/Tolerant varieties
Soybean	Rust	PK 1024, PK 1029, JS 80-21, Indira soybean 9 and MAUS 61-2
	Charcoal rot	NRC 2, NRC 37, JS 71 05, LSb 1, MACS 13 and JS 97-52
	Rhizoctonia aerial blight	PK 472, PK 1042, PK 564 and SL 295
	Anthracnose & pod blight	Bragg, Himso 1563, PK 472, JS 80-21, Pusa 37, VLS 21 and NRC 12
	Yellow mosaic	PK 416, PK 472, PS 564, PK 1024, PK 1029, PK 1042, Pusa 37, SL 295, SL 525, SL 688 and JS 97 52
	Soybean mosaic	JS 71-05, KHSb 2, LSb 1, MACS 58, MACS 124, Punjab 1 and VLS 2
Chickpea	Vascular wilt	Avrodhi, BG 212, KPG 59, BGD 72, Pusa 391, Vijay, Vishal, Rajas, BG 256, Gujrat Gram, GNG1581, GNG 1292,Virat, GJ 3, RSG88, JG315, JG74, JG11, JG322, JG63, JG12, JG14, JG16, JGK1, JGK2, JGK3, KAK2, Subhra BG 1053, HK2, JAK1 9218, Phule G9531, RSG 931, RSG 963, CSG 8962, DCP 92-3, JSC 55, JSC56, HK 05-169
	Dry root rot	JSC 37, JG 25174, CSJ 556, MPJG 89- 1155, MPJG 89- 9023, CSJ 592, Rajas, JS 2000- 07, ICCC 32, GL769
	Ascochyta blight	C235, GS43,CG558, Himachal channa1, Himachal channa 2, IPC 08-11, 23094, GNG 1581, GPF2, PBG5, Gaurav(H75-35), BG 267, Vardhan, Samrat
	Botrytis grey mould	BG 276, GL90159, GL 9-1071, GL92162, HK94-134, IPCK 2004- 29, ICC38, ICC 202, ICC1069
Pigeonpea	Phytophthora blight	BDN1, ICPL 150, ICPL 288, ICPL 304 and KPBR 80-1-4
	Sterility mosaic	ICPL 157, NP(WR)15, Bahar
Pea	Powdery mildew	Rachna, Pant P5, DMR 11, HUP 2, JP 885, KFP 103, Ambika, Shubhra, Aparna, Azad P4, Pusa Panna
	Rust	Hans, DMR 11, Type 163
Mungbean/ Urdbean	Powdery mildew	Moongbean-TARM 1, Pusa 9072 &Urdbean LBG 17
	Yellow mosaic virus	Moong bean- PDM 54 (Moti), PDM 84-139 (Samrat), PDM 84-143, PDM – 11. ML-337, Pant Moong MUM 2, MH-88-111 and MUM-2 Urd bean- Pant U 19, Pant U – 30,UG 218, PDU 1, PDU 88 -31

Crop	Name of disease	Resistant/Tolerant varieties
Mustard/ Rapeseed	White Rust	Pusa Karishma (LES-39), Jawahar Mustard-1, PBR 91
	White rust, Alternaria blight, Powdery mildew	Indian mustard-91, Toria-16, Yellow sarson-11, Gobhi sarson-11, Brown Sarson-3; Karan Rai-4, Taramira-5 and Black mustard-1
	Late blight.	Kufri Badshah, Kufri chipsona- 1, Kufri chipsona-2, Kufri frysona, Kufri chipsona- 3, Kufri chipsona- 4, Kufri frysona, Kufri, girdhari
	Early and late blight	Kufri badshah, Kufri jeevan, Kufri jyoti, Kufri kanchan, Kufri kashigaro, Kufri khyati
Tomato	Bacterial wilt	Arka Ananya, Arka Abhijit, Arka Abha, Arka Alok
	Tomato leaf curl virus	Arka Ananya, Kashi Vishesh, Kashi Amrit, COTH 2, TNAU Tomato Hybrid Co3
	Root knot nematode	Pusa-120, Pusa Hybrid-2, Pusa Hybrid-4, Arka Vardan, Hisar Lalit, TNAU Tomato Hybrid Co3
Chilli	Fusarium Wilt	Phule Jyoti, Phule Mukta
	Fruit rot	Hisar Shakti, Hisar Vijay, TNAU Chilli Hybrid Co 1
	Powdery mildew	ArkaSuphal, ArkaHarita, Arka Meghana, Hisar Shakti, Hisar Vijay, Phule Mukta
	Viral diseases and leaf curl complex	Pusa Sadabahar, Arka Harita, Arka Meghana, Arka Sweta, Hisar Shakti, Hisar Vijay, Pant C-1
Brinjal	Bacterial wilt	Pusa Purple Cluster, Pusa Anupama, Arka Anand, Arka Keshav, Arka Nidhi, ArkaNeelkanths, JC-1, JC-2, Pant Samrat, Pant Brinjal Hybrid1
	Phomopsis blight	JC-1, JC-2, Pant Samrat, Pant Brinjal Hybrid1, Azad B-2
	Little leaf virus	JC-1, JC-2
Banana	Fusarium wilt	Poovan, Robusta, Moongil
	Moko disease / Bacterial wilt	Poovan and Monthan.
	Sigatoka leaf spot	Ney Poovan, Pachanadan, Karpuravalli, Fhia 1 (Gold finger), Sannachenkadali
	Panama wilt	Dwarf Cavendish, Robusta, Fhia 1 (Gold finger), Anaikomban, NivedyaKadali.
	Bunchy top disease	Poovan, Pachanadan
Grapes	Powdery mildew	Chholth Red ,Skibba Red, Chholth white
	Downy mildew	Amber Queen, Dogridge, Red Sultana
	Anthracnose	Golden queen, Goldenmuscat, Bangalore blue
	Powdery mildew and downy mildew	Bangalore blue, Concord, Champion, Catawba

Crop	Name of disease	Resistant/Tolerant varieties
Cotton	Fuarium wilt	AK-145, Sanjay,Digvijay,LD-327,PA32
	Verticiliium wilt	MCU-5VT, Suravhi
	Leaf curl virus	H-1117, H1226,H1236, H1861,LH-2076,RS875,RS810,RS2013,LHH-144,CSHH-198,CSHH-238,CSHH-243

Advantages of HPR as a component of IDM

- Most attractive form of defense,as long as it remains effective.
- Specific to the target diseases without affecting natural enemies.
- Easily accepted and adopted by farmers.
- Provides protection at no cost to the farmers or the community.
- Increases efficacy of fungicides and natural enemies.
- Requires less frequent and low doses of fungicides.
- Some varieties have durable resistance for long periods.
- Only practical method of control of diseases like viruses, phytoplasmas wilts, and rusts etc. in which chemical control is very expensive and impractical.

Disadvantages of HPR

- **Time consuming**: Requires from 3-10 years by traditional breeding programmes to develop a resistant variety.
- **Genetic limitation**: Absence of resistance genes among available germplasm.
- **Biotype development**: A biotype is a new population capable of damaging and surviving on plants previously resistant to other population of same species.

Compatibility of HPR in IDM

a. Compatibility with chemical control

- HPR enhances efficacy of pesticides.
- Higher control of disease in resistant variety compared to susceptible variety.
- Less number of application fungicides is needed to control disease on resistant variety.
- Less chances of development of resistant in pathogen.

b. Compatibility with biological control

- Increases shelf life of resistant varieties.
- Eco friendly in nature.
- Reduces the fungicide application.

c. Compatibility with cultural method

- Establishment of a growing environment that favors the crop over the pathogen.
- Reducing plant stress through environmental modification, promotes good plant health and aids in reducing damage from some plant disease.

9.4 Biological Management

The 2020 World Population Data Sheet indicates that world population is projected to increase from 7.8 billion in 2020 to 9.9 billion by 2050. This level represents an increase of more than 25% from 2020. There is continued need for pest management in agriculture, with pressure continuously increasing on agriculture to achieve higher yield from limited or even lesser land. The excessive use of synthetic pesticides is no longer sustainable. It causes land, air and water contamination. It is also responsible for causing resistance development in pathogens and insects as well as adverse impacts on natural enemies and humans.

Thus there is need to switch for more environmentally safe and ecologically sound disease control methods such as bioagents/ biopesticides. Biopesticide is a term that has been applied with a narrow focus on preparations containing living microorganisms, through to a broader definition that encompasses botanical compounds and semiochemicals(e.g. pheromones).

Biocontrol or Biological Control

Out of the three methods of disease control *viz.*, cultural, chemical & biocontrol, biocontrol or biological control has gained popularity amongst audiences across the globe. In biocontrol, one organism controls the other with the ultimate goal of pathogen elimination for better crop growth & production in an environmental-friendly setting. It is the most technical disease management method in agriculture in which several microorganisms are introduced in the field to eliminate diseases and this method boosts soil productivity. So, is Biocontrol the future of agriculture in India?

A. Brief History

Different people have different definitions for Bio-control. The 'father' of modern-day bio-control, Prof. Harry Scott Smith defines it as the use of natural enemies, introduced or manipulated to control insect pests. While the term was first coined by prof. Harry Scott Smith in 1919, Biocontrol has been under practice for centuries. The first use of an insect species to control another insect species comes from "Nanfang Caomu Zhuang" in 304 AD, in which people sold insects to protect citrus fruits without which they could undergo heavy damage. Another instance of biocontrol was the ancient practice of changing the crop species every second or third year. Such crop rotation allowed the pest or pathogens present in the soil to decrease because,of the predatory, competitive and other antagonistic effects imposed by associated flora and fauna. Despite its use in agriculture for centuries, the technique is still in its infancy or beginning stage. Half of the farmers, still unaware of its existence continue to rely on chemical methods of eliminating diseases.

Definition of biological control

Biological control can be defined as "The action of parasites, predators or pathogens in maintaining another organism's population density at a lower average than would occur in their absence".

or

"The destruction or suppression of undesirable insects, other animals or plants by the introduction, encouragement, or artificial increase of their natural enemies".

Types of biological control

There are three types of bio logical control.

1. Partial biological control
2. Substantial biological control
3. Complete biological control

1. **Partial biological control:** If control is achieved at some what higher average population densities than it is economically satisfactory.
2. **Substantial biological control:** If biological control can be substantially successful economically for a period of time, the only partially so far a subsequent period. Here a degree of biological control is evaluated on economic yard stick.
3. **Complete biological control:** If biological agent is successful economically for a very long period of time. So far as such success has not yet been achieved. Outstanding economic feature of successful biological control is that once achieved, it is essentially permanent. Also, it does agree with man's purposeful activity.

Field of biological control

Study includes basic as well as applied aspects of natural enemies for the regulation of pest /pathogen population density.

1. Basic studies

It includes research on fundamental aspects like isolation, identification, selection of potential strain, taxonomy, biology, physiology, genetics, ecology and demography, behavior, culturing methods and nutrition.

2. Applied studies

a. Introduction of natural enemies

Purposeful introduction of new natural enemies is usually based on the fact that many, if not most, agricultural pests have been accidentally introduced into the area concerned where there indigenous natural enemies have been designed.

b. Augmentation

This phase of biological control deals with manipulation of natural enemies themselves in order to make them more efficient in the regulation of diseases and pests.

c. Conservation of natural enemies

Another approach to the enhancement of biological control would be to modify the environment in such a way that any adverse environment effect would be eliminated.

Scope of Biological Control

In the future, workers in biological control must continue to deepen and broaden their efforts, as this field has received immense enthusiastic applause during past century. These research workers showed successful practical results in more than 60 countries of the world. The partially exploited field has numerous dimension of future scope.

1. Promoting basic research

- Basic research areas in the field of biology, ecology, systematics, biochemistry, population dynamics etc. have enormous contributing value to biological suppression which needs to be studied.
- There is lot of scope to intensify the studies in these areas which can improve and synergize the biological control .
- This study would help genuinely in the application of IDM strategies of the disease.

2. Scope to exploit the bioagent on crop disease

- Biocontrol assumes significance considering the resolve of many states in India to go completely organic.
- There are many successful biocontrol agents that have been tested and commercialized in India.
- Farm yard manure (FYM) enriched with Trichoderma a and Pseudomonas are used to control soil borne diseases.
- Bioformulation of Kalisena (*Aspergillus niger* based formulation) and Josh (VAM based formulation) are also found to be effective in managing wilt infections in Indian conditions..

3. Help to reduce pollution hazards

- The biocontrol agents are based either on plant parts / plant products, microorganisms such as bacteria, viruses and fungi, fungal and bacterial enzymes, enzyme inhibitors, antibiotics that play an important role in control of plant-pathogenic fungi .
- Utilization of bioagent can help in establishment of population regulation process of serious pests by reducing the load of toxic pesticides and their side effects.

4. Necessity to intensify new horizons of biological control

- Use of fungal bioagents, parasitoids and predators is popular concept of biological control, which gave good success in several cases.
- Similarly new trends such as use of biotypes, strains, hybrids of parasites, use of novel biopesticides like entomogenous fungi, viruses, nematodes are to be search properly and its harmonious use in disease suppression needs to be exploited.

5. Adoption of biological control methods in agro industries

- Although use of bioagent has many benefits but there is need to adjust with other methods like chemical control of disease.
- The pesticides should be less toxic to natural enemies and needs to be identified and employed in disease suppression.
- Biological control helps in maintaining 'Balance of Nature' as it is the phase of natural control.

Differences between disease bio-control and insect bio-control

The biological control of plant diseases differs from insect biocontrol in following ways.

Differences between disease bio-control and insect bio-control

Sl.No	Disease bio-control	Insect bio-control
1	Disease control is mainly achieved by antibiosis, competition and by hyperparasites	Mainly by parasites and predators.
2	Antagonists are mainly passive and are not mobile. Contact of pathogen is accidental.	Parasites are active, mobile and seek their prey.
3	It is a mass effect. For a single species of pathogen a large number of antagonists / competitors available	Single predator / parasite for single prey.
4	This method relies mainly on native organisms.	Introduction of parasites / predators from other countries are normally followed.
5	Pathogen free seeds and planting materials are widely used.	Pest free seeds are not used.

How biocontrol works

The agents of biocontrol include- pests or disease agents, natural enemies, and plants or animals immunized to protect themselves. Some of the approaches to biocontrol include:

1. A classical approach involving the regulation of pest population through other microorganisms.

2. Exclusionary method of protection in which a living layer of protecting microorganisms is plastered on the plants and animals to deter infection.
3. Resistance and immunization approach or systems of self-defense.

The success of biocontrol method depends upon knowledge of biological interactions with the ecosystem, cellular organisms and molecular levels.

The complexities of biocontrol make it unpopular in comparison with cultural or chemical prevention methods. But, this method is more stable, effective and long lasting.

Unlike other methods, biocontrol has a clear past, with no evidence of any negative effects of biocontrol agents on the environment.

The different mechanisms of antagonism occur across a spectrum of directionality related to the amount of inter species contact and specificity of the interactions is mentioned below.

Types of inter species antagonisms leading to biological control of plant pathogens

Type	Mechanism	Examples
Direct antagonism	Hyperparasitism/ predation	Lytic/some nonlytic myco viruses *Ampelomyces quisqualis* *Lysobacteren zymogenes* *Pasteuria penetrans* *Trichoderma virens*.
Mixed-path antagonism	Antibiotics	2,4-diacetylphloroglucin Phenazines Cyclic lipopeptides
	Lytic enzymes	Chitinases Glucanases Proteases.
	Unregulated waste products	Ammonia Carbon dioxide Hydrogen cyanide.
	Physical/chemical interference	Blockage of soil pores Germination signals consumption Molecular cross-talk confused.
Indirect antagonism	Competition	Exudates/leachates consumption Siderophore scavenging Physical niche occupation.
	Induction of host resistance	Contact with fungal cell walls Detection of pathogen-associated molecular patterns Phytohormone-mediated induction.

Role of biocontrol

1. Disease control

- *Trichoderma* is a potential biocontrol agent and used extensively for post harvest disease control.
- It has been used successfully against various pathogenic fungi belonging to various genera, *viz,Fusarium*, *Phytophthora,Sclerotia.*

2. Plant growth promoter

- Biocontrol agents solublize phosphates and micronutrients.
- The application of biocontrol *viz Trichodem/Pseudomons* with plants such as grasses increases the number of deep roots, thereby increasing the plant's ability to resist drought.

3. Stimulation of plant resistance and plant defense mechanism

- Species of *Trichoderma* or *Pseudomonas* added to the rhizosphere protect plants against numerous classes of pathogens including viral, bacterial and fungal,
- It points to the induction resistance mechanisms similar to the hypersensitive response (HR), systemic acquired resistance (SAR), and induced systemic resistance (ISR) in plants.

4. Transgenic plants

- Introduction of endochitinase gene from *Trichoderma* into plants such as tobacco and potato plants increased their resistance to fungal growth.
- Selected transgenic lines are highly tolerant to foliar pathogens such as *Alternaria alternata*, *A. solani,* and *Botrytis cinerra* as well as to the soil borne pathogen, *Rhizoctonia* spp.

5. Bioremediation

- *Trichoderma* strains play an important in the bioremediation of soil that are contaminated with pesticides and herbicides.
- They have the ability to degrade a wide range of insecticides: organocholorines, organophosphates and carbamates.

Advantages of biological control

Advantages

- Gives protection to the crop throughout the crop period.
- Highly effective against specific plant diseases.
- They do not cause toxicity to the plants.
- Easy to handle and apply to the target.

- Safer to the environment and to the person who applies them.
- Multiply easily in the soil and leave no residual problem.
- Eliminate pathogens from the site of infection.
- Biocontrol agents can be combined with biofertilizers.
- Cheaper than other methods.

Disadvantages

- Used only against specific diseases.
- They are less effective than the fungicides.
- Have slow effect in the control of plant diseases.
- They are mostly unavailable in larger quantities.
- Preventive in nature.
- Requires skilled persons to handle.
- Shelf life of biocontrol agents is short.
- Quality need to be checked at periodical interval and should be maintained at required level for effective use.
- Efficiency of biocontrol agents is mainly decided by environmental conditions.
- Biocontrol agent under certain circumstances may beomce a pathogen.

What is *Trichoderma*?

- *Trichoderma*, genus of asexually reproducing fungi.
- It is present in nearly all tropical and temperate soils.
- Strains of Trichoderma spp. are strong opportunistic invaders, fast growing, prolific producers of spores and powerful antibiotic producers.
- These properties make these fungi ecologically very successful and are the reason for their ubiquitousness.
- They show a high level of genetic diversity.
- Trichoderma can be used to produce a wide range of products of commercial and ecological interest.
- Most common BCAs of the Trichoderma genus are strains of *T. viride*, *T. virens* and *T. harzianum.* Several plant diseases caused by fungi can be potentially controlled by Trichoderma species.

Importamt plant diseases controlled by *Trichoderma* species

Name of the disease	Disease causing organism	Name of the crop
Collar rot	*Sclerotium rolfsii*	Elephant foot yam
Damping off	*Pythium, Phytopthora, Fusarium*	Chilli, Tomato, Brinjal
Rhizome rot	*Pythium, Phytopthora, Fusarium*	Ginger, Onion
Wilt	*Fusarium oxysporum*	Tomato, Brinjal
Sheath blight	*Rhizoctonia solani*	Maize, Rice

Secret of success of *Trichoderma* as BCAs

The success of *Trichoderma* strains as BCAs is due to their

- High reproductive capacity.
- Ability to survive under very unfavorable conditions.
- Efficiency in the utilization of nutrient.
- Capacity to modify the rhizosphere.
- Strong aggressiveness against phyto pathogenic fungi.
- Efficiency in promoting plant growth and defense mechanisms.

Method of application of *Trichodema*

The biological control practices of the plant pathogens start with the definite principles and practices. There is no hazard to flora, fauna and life and also no disturbance to soil , water and air on account of biological control practices. The following practices are taken up in biological control of the plant diseases.

1. Seed treatment

- Seed treatment with *Trichoderma* has tremendous potential to make the control a great success especially for seed and seedling diseases in vegetables, fruit, forest and other plantation crop nurseries .
- *Trichoderma* seed treatment increased plant stand, reduced seedling mortality and are effective as the chemical fungicides.
- Generally seed treatment with talc based *Trichoderma* product @ 4gm/kg of seed is recommended for control of root diseases of crop plants.

2. Soil application

- The talc based formulations of *Trichoderma* are used as soil application by mixing in well decomposed compost before application into soil.
- The quantity required is high and varies from 125-250 kg/ha.
- It is mixed with, FYM and broadcast on the soil and then incorporated into soil through harrowing.
- It is used to control Fusarium wilt , Sclerotium foot rots and Macrophomina root rots. Applied at least 2 weeks before sowing of crops.

3. Furrow application

- It is comparatively economical to broadcasting and is followed in nurseries. The quantity required is 130-160 kg/ha.
- It should be applied in the open furrows and then covered with the soil. Applied 15 days before sowing of the seeds.

4. Root zone application

- This is used in wide spaced crops such as plantation and fruit crops.
- The formulation is mixed in soil in the root zone upto one kg/plant.

5. Wound treatment

- This is used to treat pruning wounds of forest and plantation crops.
- It is done in peach and plum against silver leaf disease.

6. Pot culture treatment

- This treatment is generally applicable in nurseries .
- Application of bioagents @ 5gm/kg of soil is recommended.

7. Seedling treatment

- The seedling are dispersed in the solution of *Trichoderma* and then they are taken for sowing to control the seedling blight diseases.

8. Spraying

- The liquid suspension prepared by mixing powder and water to get 10^6-10^8 cfu /ml .
- It should be sprayed on to the plant surface and soil surface at the rte of 4g/ liter of water.

Plant Growth Promoting Rhizobacteria (PGPR)

- The rhizosphere bacteria that can colonize the plant roots have been termed as rhizobacteria by Kloepper and Schroth (1978).
- The rhizobacteria that are strains of *Pseudomonas fluorescens* and *Pseudomonas putida*, have been regarded to have coevolved with their host plants.
- The term rhizobacteria has been used to accentuate their intimate association with root.
- These naturaly occurring, non pathogenic, root colonizing bacteria, may be harmful or beneficial for growth of plants are called deleterious rhizobacteria (DRB) and plant growth promoting rhizobacteria (PGPR), respectively.
- PGPR, fall under genera Pseudomonas, Bacillus, Arthrobactor, Achromobacter, Citrobactor, Enterobacter and Flavobacterium.
- PGPR besides enhancing growth and yields, are also potential biocontrol agents and are usually isolated from suppressive soils.
- Most of the PGPR are fluorescent pseudomonas (*Pseudomonas fluorescens* and *Pseudomonas putida*) but also include non fluorescent *Pseudomonas* sp., *Bacillus subtilis* and *Serratia* spp.

Ways that PGPR promote plant growth

- Increasing nitrogen fixation in legumes.
- Promoting free-living nitrogen-fixing bacteria.
- Increasing supply of other nutrients, such as phosphorus, sulphur, iron and copper.
- Producing plant hormones.
- Enhancing other beneficial bacteria or fungi.
- Controlling fungal and bacterial diseases.
- Controlling insect pests.

Application of PGPRs

Effectiveness of PGPRs does not depend only on suitable PGPRs strains but also on suitable methods and strategies for introducing and maintaining the organisms in crops.Most of the PGPRs strains are usually applied as:

1. Soil application
2. Seed coating
3. Foliar spray

1. Soil application

- The granule formulation of the PGPR strain has been developed specially for the soil application.
- Sometimes it can be placed near the root zone along the seedlings during transplanting.

2. Seed coating

- The application of PGPR strain is quite convenient, as little amount of inoculums is required to disperse it along the seed surface.
- Seed coating /bacterization is recommended to those PGPR strain, which have sufficient rhizosphere competence so that they may proliferate easily in rhizosphere , increased to sufficient number to express the biocontrol and growth promoting potentiality.
- The agents like Pseudomonas or Bacillus are applied through seed bacterization.
- Seed treatment may be given as dry seed treatment, wet seed treatment and slurry seed treatment.

3. Foliar application

- The foliar application of PGPR strain is comparatively less common as compared to seed or soil application.

- However, for the biocontrol of certain aerial plant pathogens the wet formulation is suspended and applied through sprayng in case of bocontrol of bacterial blight of rice.

Precaution

- Formulation of PGPR should be purchased from an authorized /recommended company shop or retailer.
- The date of manufacturing and expiry of utilization must be verified before delivery.
- During storage packets should not be exposed to direct sunlight and should also not be stored with chemical fertilizers and pesticides.
- Formulation should be stored in cool, and dry place.
- The entire contents of the pack should be used at one time.

Biopesticides

- Biologically based products are often referred to as "biorationals" or "biopesticides".
- Biorational is used in broad reference to any biologically based product used in agriculture that includes fertilizers, pesticides, herbicides, plant growth regulators, and various other products.
- A biopesticides is defined by the U.S. Environmental Protection Agency (EPA) as a pesticide derived from natural materials.
- A compound that kills organisms by virtue of specific biological effects rather than as a broader chemical poison.
- Differ from biocontrol agents in being passive agents, where as biocontrol agents actively seek the pest.
- The rationale behind replacing conventional pesticides with biopesticides is that the latter are more likely to be selective and biodegradable."

Classification of Biopesticides

Biopesticides fall into three major classes:

1. Microbial pesticides:
2. Biochemical pesticides
3. Plant incorporated protectants (PIPs):

1. Microbial pesticides

- Contains microorganism as the main active ingredients that function as biological control agents, affecting the pathogen directly or indirectly through the compounds they produce or by stimulating specific plant responses.

- It consist of bacteria, entomopathogenic fungi_or viruses (and sometimes includes the metabolites that bacteria or fungi produce).
- Entomopathogenic nematodes are also often classed as microbial pesticides, even though they are multi-cellular.

2. Biochemical pesticides

- Naturally occurring substances that control pests by non toxic mechanisms.
- Substances that control diseases in this category include potassium bicarbonate, hydrogen dioxide, phosphorus acids, plant extracts, and botanicals

3. Plant incorporated protectants (PIPs)

- Least common type of biopesticide.
- These are pesticidal substances produced by plants that contains genetic material added to the plant often through genetic engineering.(e.g GM crops)

Difference between biopesticde and chemical pesticide

Biopesticides	Chemical pesticides
These do not harm non target species	Non-target species are also harmed
They do not pollute the environment	Cause pollution; sometimes serious
No harmful residues remain in food, fodder and fibers	Harmful residues may often remain in food, fodder and fibers
Relatively cheaper	Relatively costlier
Insects are expected not to develop resistance to biopesticides	Insects may become resistant, e.g., Heliothis has become resistant to most insecticides
Since they are highly specific, correct identification of the pest is essential	It is often not critical
High specificity may often make the use of two or more biopesticides necessary	Often not required
Performance may be variable due to the influence of biotic and abiotic factors of the environment	This is not often the case

Commercialization of biopesticides

- Thirty four microorganisms have been permitted by CIB for agriculture production .
- Only five viz.,Trichoderma viride, Trichoderma harzianum, Pseudomonas fluorescens Beauveria bassiana and Ampelomyces quisqualis are used for the managmment of plant diseases.
- Trichoderma is most exploited and have many success stories in India.
- Commericalization of biocontrol products is a multi-step process involving a wide range of activities.
- The commercial success of biocontrol agents requires

1. Consistant and broad spectrum action

2. Easy availability of carrier materials
3. Longer shelf life
4. Safety and stability
5. Low capital costs.
6. Economical and viable market demand.

Steps in commercialization

1. Isolation of antagonist
2. Screening of antagonist
3. Pot test and field efficacy
4. Mass production
5. Fermentation
6. Formulation
7. Toxicology
8. Industrial linkages
9. Quality control
10. Registration of bioagents

1. Isolation of antagonist

- Isolation of an effective bioagents plays an important role in disease management.
- Isolation is done from the pathogen suppressive soils either by baiting the soil with fungal structures like sclerotia of pathogen or dilution plate technique .
- Isolate location specific and crop specific isolates and establish consortium of biocontrol agents .
- It could be used for the development of mixtures of biocontrol agents suited for different ecological niche.

2. Screening of antagnoist

- Selection of an effective strain decides the viability of the technology.
- Strains isolated from the diverse cropping system have to be ascertained for its virulence and broad spectrum of action against diverse pathogens causing serious economic threat to cultivation.
- A proper yardstick should be developed to screen to antagonistic potentiality of the biocontrol agents.
- Once effective strains have been identified with the *in vitro* assays , a further selection must be done by studying other factors like:
    - Specificity i.e strain should be inactive against crops and beneficial organisms.

- Tolerance to low or high temperature .
- Strain should have the ability to secrete increased level of cell wall lytic enzymes (glucanases, chitinases and celluloses), antibiotic and plant growth promotion.
- Interactions with other Trichoderma strains already present in the cropping systems.
- Compatibility with agrochemicals used in the crop.
- Shelf life and inoculum efficacy under commercial conditions.
- Activity *in vivo* using experimentally induced diseases on plants.
- Suitability for formulation as foliar sprays and/or soil enhancements .
- Long-term survival in field conditions.

A yard stick should be developed comprising of above mentioned components. Each component should be given weightage depending upon their role in disease management.

3. Pot test and field efficacy

- The pathogen, antagonists and plant are coexposed to controlled environmental conditions.
- Host should be exposed to heavy inoculums pressure of the pathogen along with the antagonist.
- This will provide ecological data on the performance of the antagonist under controlled conditions.
- Promising antagonists selected from controlled environment are further tested for their efficacy under field conditions along with the standard recommended fungicides.
- Trials on field efficacy should be conducted for at least 15 to 20 locations under diverse environmental conditions to promote the best candidate for mass multiplication and formulation development.

4. Mass production and formulation development

Mass production is achieved through solid and liquid fermentation techniques.

a. Solid fermentation techniques

- Commonly used medium : Cheap cereal grains like, sorghum, millets, ragi etc.
- Carrier used for microbial growth: Insoluble materials in water

b. Liquid fermentation techniques

- Commonly used medium : Potato dextrose broth, V -8 juice, Molasses-yeast medium and Wheat bran
- Carrier used for microbial growth: soluble materials in water

- Liquid formulation is emerging as the way forward for cost effective, eco-friendly and sustainable agriculture.
- Capacity to replace the traditional chemical pesticides and carrier-based solid biopesticides

Advantages of liquid formulation

- Offer longer shelf life (up to 2 years).
- Carrier-free activity.
- Ease in handling and application.
- Convenience in storage and transport.
- Easy quality control.
- Enhanced export potential.
- Reduces frequency of application.
- Decreases cost of plant protection.

Comparative technical analysis

Features	Liquid biopesticide formulations	Solid biopesticide formulations	Chemical Pesticides
Safety (non target pests)	Safe	Safe	Hazardous
Efficacy spectrum (target pests)	Broad	Broad	Narrow
Host Resistance	Low	Low	High
Shelf life	High	Moderate	High
Portability	High	Medium	Low
Contaminants	Negligible	Moderate	--
Persistence vs sustainability	Sustainable	Sustainable	Persist
Additional benefit	PGP	PGP	--
Rate of application	Low	Low	high

5. Formulation

Blending of active ingredients like fungal spores with the inert mmaterial to alter the physical characteristics of to a more desirable form id called formulation. A final formulation should have following characteristics:

- Be easy to handle.
- Be stable over a range of -5 to 35°C.
- Shelf life of two years at room temperature.
- Product should have minimum shelf life of 8 to 12 months for industrialization.
- Researches concentrated to increase the shelf life of the formulation .

Characteristics of an ideal formulation

i) Increased shelf life.

ii) Not phytotoxic to the crop plants.

iii) Tolerate adverse environmental conditions.
iv) Cost effective and should give reliable control of plant diseases.
v) Dissolve well in water.
vi) Carriers must be cheap and readily available for formulation development.
vii) Compatible with other agrochemicals.

Improvement of formulation efficacy

- Development of compatible consortia.
- Adjuvants, spreaders and stickers.
- Mutation.
- Genetic recombination.
- Protoplast fusion.
- Molecular approaches.

6. Industrial linkages

- The initial discovery of an effective antagonist, genetic manipulation of antagonist to develop superior strains and studies on mechanisms, field efficacy and protocols for the development of formulation are carried out by the research institutes.
- The partnership between the institutes and stakeholders is needed to take this technology to the entire country.
- Corporates resources are needed for the large scale production, toxicology, wide range field testing, registration and marketing.
- Entrepreneurship means exchange of intellectual property for research grants, and a royalty stream with the establishment of University-Industry partnership for the benefit of both.
- Entreprenuership needed a patent application on the strain and the related technology, particularly on the efficacy data, identity of the organism, toxicological data and delivery system.
- Ideally, the process of entrepreneurship will result in an academic corporate research team working towards a common goal.

7. Registration of biocontrol agents

- Bio-pesticides have been put under Indian Insecticide Act 1968.
- Registration of the bio pesticides has become mandatory before it is commercialized .

Basic information required on the product for registration

- Systematic name: Genus and species.
- Common name, if any.

- Natural occurrence- morphological description.
- Manufacturing process- solid or liquid state fermentation.
- Qualitative analysis.
- Toxicity & residual analysis.
- CFU on selective medium.
- Absence of Gram –ve bacterial contaminants (*Salmonella, Shigella and Vibrio*).
- Moisture content.
- Shelf life claim- two different location along with meteorological data.

8. Quality control

- This is very much obligatory to retain the confidence of the farmers on the efficacy of biocontrol agents.
- Being the living organisms, their population in a product influences the shelf life.
- The population load of the antagonists decides the minimum level of requirement for bringing the effective biological control of the plant diseases.

CFU count & Shelf life

- Data required for claiming one year shelf life of the product.
- Microbe should remain viable for 15 months.
- CFU count not less than 2×10^6 spores/ml or g.
- The pathogenic contaminants such as *Salmonella, Shigella and Vibrio* should not be present.
- Other microbial contaminants not to exceed 1×10^4 counts per ml or g.

Moisture content

- Maximum moisture content of the product should not exceed more than 8 per cent for dry formulation of fungi and 12 per cent for bacteria.

Toxicology

- It includes information of antagonist on safety to men, plants, animals and soil microflora.
- Toxicology studies have to be done separately for each and every biocontrol organism.
- Biopesticides are regulated in an appropriate way to confirm the international standards.
- Safety and environmental considerations could not be taken for grante.
- Huge investment on toxicological studies warrants for the linkages between research organizations and stakeholders

Bioefficacy

Lab bioefficacy test

- Product should be tested against target pathogen at one of the laboratories of ICAR/SAUs/CSIR/ICMR system.
- Efficacy of promising antagonists from controlled environment are tested for its efficacy under field conditions along with the standard recommended fungicides.
- Generate ecological data on the performance of the antagonist under controlled conditions.

Field bioefficacy

- Trials on the field efficacy conducted for at least 15 to 20 locations under diverse conditions to promote the best candidate for mass multiplication and formulation development.
- Intended product should be tested for field bioefficacy under Indian conditions.
- Exposure of the host to the heavy inoculums pressure of the pathogen along with the biopesticide.

Strategies to promote commercialization

The strategies to commercialized biocontrol are

a. Popularization of biocontrol agents

- Publicity.
- Field demonstrations.
- Farmers days.
- Bio village adoption and conducting periodical trainings for commercial producers and farmers.

b. Industrial linkages

- Technical support made available to entrepreneurs on quality control and registration.
- Regular monitoring to maintain the quality.
- Constant research support to standardize the dosage, storage, and delivery systems.

Constraints to commercialization

- Paucity of correct screening protocol for the selection of promising bioagents.
- Dearth of sufficient knowledge on the microbial ecology of bioagents and pathogens.

- Optimization of fermentation and mass production technology of bioagents.
- Inconsistent performance and poor shelf life.
- Paucity of patent protection.
- Paucity of multi disciplinary approach.
- Technology constraints.
- Prohibitive registration cost.
- Awareness, training and education shortfalls.

Microbial Consortium

- A microbial consortium or consortium, is two or more microbial groups living symbiotically.
- Consortiums can be endosymbiotic or ectosymbiotic.
- The concept of a consortium was first introduced by Johannes Reinke in 1872.

Advantages

- Robustness.
- Efficiency.
- Modularity.

Mode of action of microbial consortia

- Antibiosis.
- Competition.
- Mycoparasitism.
- Additive or Synergistic effect.
- Induced systemic resistance.

Essential for success of microbial consortia

- Compatibility of microbial components.
- Synergism of microbial components.

Various applications of microbial consortia

- Bio-control agents.
- Bio fertilizers.
- Rhizosphere bioremediation of pesticides.
- Effective degradation of organic wastes.
- Reclamation of soils.

Examples

Product/Trade name	Species/strain of *Trichoderma*	Agency/Company
Bioderma	*Trichoderma viride+ Trichoderma harzianum*	*Fusarium, Botryosphaeria,*
Ecoderma	*Trichoderma viride+ Trichoderma harzianum*	*Rhizoctonia, Pythium, Phytophthora*
Binap- T&W	*Trichoderma harzianum+ T. polysporum*	Wood decay fungi

Biocontrol is the need of the hour

- The way electric, non-polluting vehicles are replacing the harmful fossil fuel-powered vehicles, Biocontrol too will balance the chemical method of pest prevention.
- Biocontrol is one of the most popular methods to meet India's agricultural requirements in the future.
- It's an economical and more environmentally friendly approach to meet our agricultural needs.
- But a lot of work, research and time is needed to make Biocontrol the first preference of every Indian farmer.
- With the right investment in R&D and production, the need can be met efficiently.
- Biocontrol is the current need of the hour, not only for the soil but for humans as well as the environment!

9.5 Legislative Management

Plant Quarantine

- The term 'Quarantine' is derived from the Latin word quarantum, meaning 40.
- It refers to the 40 days period of detention of ships from countries with bubonic plague and cholera in the Middle Ages.
- The first such quarantine was imposed in Venice in 1374.Present quarantine laws now include plants.
- Plant quarantine, restrict entry of plants, plant products, soil, cultures of living organisms, packing materials, and commodities, as well as their containers and means of conveyance to protect agriculture and the environment from avoidable damage by hazardous organisms.
- They exclude dangerous organisms while permitting plants and plant products to enter.
- The term exclusion convey this objective more clearly than plant quarantine.
- Exclusion relates to keeping organisms out.

- Plant quarantine relates to keeping plants out.
- 'Plant Quarantine' is an endeavour through which restrictions are imposed by the govenment to regulate the introduction and movement of plants and plant materials with a view to prevent introduction of exotic pests /pathogens into uninfested areas.The term frequently used in plant quarantine are *hazard, risk*, and *safeguards*.
- **Hazard**: is the danger that a specified pathogen is known or perceived to present to the agriculture of the importing country gain entry on imported items and subsequently become established.
- **Risks**: is the chance that a hazardous organism will enter and become established.
- **Safeguards**: are action taken to reduce the risk of introducing hazardous organisms.

Pests introduced in India

Pests	Sicentific Name	Year of Intorudction
Lantana weed	*Lantana camara*	1809
Coffee rust	*Hemilia vastatrix*	1879
Late blight of potato	*Phytophthora infestans*	1883
Wooly apple aphid	*Eriosomala nigerum*	1889
Grape downy mildew	*Plasmopara viticola*	1910
San Jose Scale	*Quadrapidiotus perniciosus*	1911
Water hyacinth	*Eichhornia crassies*	1914
Potato tuber moth	*Phthorimaeao perculella*	1937
Banana bunchy top virus		1940
Wart of potato	*Synchytrium endobioticum*	1953
Congress grass	*Parthenium hysterophorus*	1956
Golden nematodes	*Globodera rostochiensis & G pllida*	1961
Apple scab	*Venturia inaequalis*	1978
Downy mildew of sunflower	*Plasmopara halstedii*	1984
Peanut stripe virus		1987
Sunflower necrosis	*Sunflower necrosis virus*	1997
Cotton mealy bug	*Phenococcus solenopsis*	2006
Papaya mealy bug	*Paracoccus marginatus*	2009
Tomato leaf minor	*Tutaabosoluta meyrick*	2014
Root knot nematode	*Meloidogyne enterolobii*	2016
White rust of chrysanthemum	*Puccinia horiana*	2016
Fall armyworm in maize	*Spodoptera frugiperda*	2018

Importance

- The importance of plant quarantine has increased because of the increase in exchange of seeds or grains for consumption along with better means of transportation.

- The international exchange of plants or their parts is practiced widely to improve crops of a country and their genetic base.
- In addition, shiploads of grains for consumption or large quantities of seeds for direct sowing are imported in many countries.
- Even minute quantities of soil and plant debris contaminating true seeds can disseminate pathogens.
- The entry of single pests and their establishment in the new environment continues to cause stern national loss till it brought under effectual control.
- In some cases a nation has to spend a few millions rupees before success in manageing the introduced pests is achieved.

Losses due to introduced plant diseases

Disease	Host	Country	Introduced From	Losses Caused
Bunchy top	Banana	India	Sri Lanka	Rs.4 crores
Wart	Potato	India	Netherland	2500 acres infected
Canker	Citrus	U.S.A	Japan	$ 13 million; 19.5 million trees destroyed
Dutch elm	Elm	U.S.A.	Holland	$ 25 million -$ 50,000 million disease
Powdery mildew	Grapevine	France	U.S.A	80% in wine production
Downy mildew	Grapevine	France	U.S.A	$ 50,000 million
Bunchy top	Banana	India	Sri Lanka	Rs. 4 crores
Wart	Potato	India	Netherlands	2500 acres infected
Blue mould	Tobacco	Europe	U.K	$ 50 million

Aim of plant quarantine

To prevent the introduction of dangerous diseases and pests or new races of a pathogen and their spread within the country.

The goal of regulatory actions are

- To delay or prevent entry of the pathogen along manmade pathways.
- If entry succeeds, to prevent infection.
- If infection succeeds, to prevent establishment of pathogens entering on manmade and natural pathways.
- If established, to minimize or retard spread.

Basic principles of plant quarantine

- The basic principles of plant quarantine is to check the entry and spread of potentially dangerous plant pathogens and insects imported along with the germplasm.

Prerequisites of Plant Quarantine Regulations

- Only pathogens and pest that pose a threat to major crops or forest should be taken into considerations.
- Formulated to control or prevent the pests and not to hinder trade or attainment of other objectives.
- Derived from adequate legislation and operated solely under the law.
- Modified as conditions change or further facts become available.
- Those responsible for quarantine measures should be properly trained and experienced.
- Professional workers and the public must co-operate on an international scale for effective operation of quarantine regulations.

Components of plant quarantine

Plant protection and quarantine (PPQ) programs, or the plant health or quarantine services in most countries, usually have three components

1. Exclusion of pathogens and pests of quarantine and economic significance that might unintentionally be moved along manmade pathways when articles are imported, or induction of the risk of introducing such hazardous organisms to an acceptance level.
2. Containment, suppression, and eradication of exotic pathogens and pests recently introduced along natural and manmade pathways.
3. Assistance to exporters of plant products, such as fruits, vegetables, plants, cut flowers, commodities, etc., in meeting the quarantine or exclusion requirements of importing countries and , therefore, based on plant health, biologically facilitating the acceptance of imports.

1. Pest Risk Analysis

Pest risk defines the chances that a pathogen or pest of quarantine significance will enter along a manmade pathway. Risk often is expressed as low, medium or intermediate, and high.

- **Low risk:** means that there is little chance that the pathogen or pest will enter.
- **High risk:** means that chances are high that the pathogen or pest could enter.
- **Acceptable risk:** An acceptable risk level means that the benefits derived after taking risk are high enough to justify taking the risk, with safe guards , in the first place.

The rules and regulations governing seed entry should be based on a matching of risk with entry decisions. If the risk is low, the entry should be liberal; if risk is high, the entry status should be conservative: and when the risk is unknown, quarantine officer need to be policy of an importing countries might prohibit all plants of high risk and by doing so take no risk, but at the cost of receiving no benefits from crop improvement.

2. Movement of pathogens

- Plant pests of quarantine importance can move along with natural and man made pathways.
- It depending upon the life cycle of the organism, the environment through which it moves, and human activities.
- At the end of the pathway, the establishment of a a pathogen or pest in a new area depend on the level of inoculums or pest carried by seeds, the susceptibility of host crop(s), and the environment.
- Exchange of germplasm creates the risk of introducing pathogens or pests of quarantine importance.
- The considerations are two fold; that exotic organisms or more virulent strains of existing ones might be introduced.
- Quarantine regulations to prevent movement of feces derived products as a potential source of introduction should be considered .
- Viable teliospores of *T.caries, T. indica* and *T. controversa* are present in feces of chickens, grasshoppers and cow.
- Hence quarantine established to prevent movement of spore contaminated seeds may miss an important avenue of potential introduction by animal and animal product movements

3. Legal basis of plant quarantine

Quarantines are regulations promulgated by governments to reduce the risk of introducing hazardous pathogens and pests on articles, including seeds from foreign countries. The legal basis of quarantine comprises

- Legislation enacted by national and sometimes state or provincial governments.
- Enabling legislation that directs the Minister of Agriculture to issue necessary rules, orders or directives.
- Legislation by a regional parliament representing groups of countries.
- The legal umbrella that covers international plant quarantine matters is the International Plant Protection Covention of 1951 (Rome Certificate). Most countries either are signitories of the Rome Convention or follow its mandates.

4. Requirement for a quarantine program

- A phytosanitory certificate that attests to the inspection, origin and identification of the seeds.
- A permit requirement for added declaration on the phytosanitory certificate that the mother plants were inspected during the growing season.

- A requirement for treatment at origin.
- The acceptance of a special certification or safe guarding program at origin, such as may be practiced at International Agricultural Research Centers (IARC)
- Inspection and treatment , if necessary ,upon arrival at port of entry.
- Isolation, special testing, or additional quarantine after entry.

National and International Regulations

- The first plant quarantine law was passed in 1873 in Germany to prohibit importation of plants and plant products from the United States to prevent the introduction of the Colorado potato beetle.
- In 1975, France imposed measures against the American pest.
- In 1877, United Kingdom Destructive Insects Act prevented the introduction and spread of this beetle.
- In 1891, first plant quarantine measure was initiated in the United States by setting up a seaport inspection station at San Pedro, CA.
- In 1912, first U.S. quarantine law was passed.
- In 1909, Federal Plant Quarantine Service was established in Australia.
- In 1914, Destructive Insects and Pest Act was passed in India.
- In 1971, Government of Greece prohibited introduction of rice seeds for sowing infected with *P. oryzae.*
- In 1980, Phillipine government introduced seed health testing plants of rice for *P. oryzae.*in addition to field inspections for breeder and foundation seeds.

On a global basis, the first International Plant Protection Convention (the Phyllozera Convention) was signed in 1881 with the objective of preventing the spread of severe pests. This convention was amended in 1889,1929 and 1951. The International Plant Protection Convention (IPPC or Rome Convention) under the Food and Agriculture Organization was established to prevent the introduction and spread of diseases and pests through legislation and organizations across international boundaries. This convention provided a model phytosanitary certificate (Rome certificate) to be adopted by member countries. Within this convention, ten regional plant protection organizations have been established on the basis of biogeographical areas

- The European and Mediterranean Plant Protection Organization (EPPO).
- The Inter-African Phytosanitary Council (IAPSC).
- Organismo International Regional de SanidadAgropecnario (OIRSA).
- The Plant Protection Committee for, the South East Asia and Pacific region. (SEAPPC).
- Near East Plant Protection Commission (NEPPC).
- Comit'e Interamericano de Protection Agricola. (CIPA).
- The Caribbean Plant Protection Commission (CPPC).

- The North American Plant Protection Organization (NAPPO).
- OrganismoBolivariano de SanidadAgropecuria (OBSA).
- Association of South East Asian Countries (ASEAN).

The regional organizations are concerned with the co ordination of lcgislation and regulations within their area, agreement on the quarantine objects, inspection procedures, etc.

Criteria for determining organisms for quarantine significance

1. General criteria

The following are general criteria considered for an organism of plant quarantine significance:

- The organism does not occur in the country but is known to cause economic damage elsewhere.
- The organism occurs in the country but is not extensively spread in the ecological range of its host in that country; is under a national domestic suppression or eradication programme; has exotic strains of quarantine importance that do not occur in the country; and/or causes economic damage or has a potential to cause such damage on economically important crops.
- The organism is a general pathogens established in the importing country. But government regulations require that commercial growers use pathogen-tested seed stocks so that imported stocks meet domestic standards.

2. Criteria based primarily on pathogen characteristics

The criteria are based on the general characteristics of a pathogen.

- Able to survive and move easily in international trade.
- Capable of developing a high population in a short time.
- Difficult to detect by general inspection or field survey.
- Capable of damaging and / or reproducing on many hosts.
- Has a potential for rapid dispersal , especially along manmade pathways.
- Has a potential for significant reduction in the quality and quantity of crop yields.
- Capable of adversely affecting the environment.

Problems in plant quarantines

Quarantine serves as a filter against the introduction of dangerous pathogens, however pathogens are still introduced. Probable reasons are that

- Difficult to detect all types of infectious pathogens by conventional methods.
- Methods may not be sensitive enough to detect traces of infection.

- Latent infections may pass undetected under post entry quarantine.
- Destruction of all infected or suspected material.
- Sensitive methods for testing fungicide treated seeds may be lacking.

Organisms of quarantine significance

Organisms of quarantine significance may include any pathogen or pest that a government (or inter governmental organization) considers to pose a threat to the agriculture and environment of the country or region. Such organism generally are exotic to that country or region but may include exotic strains or races of domestic strains.

Plant quarantine methods

The plant quarantine methods which are used individually or jointly to retard or prevent the introduction and establishment of exotic pests are;

1	Complete embargoes	• Most effective masure to exclude specific plant and products completely from a country infected with highly destructive pests • Or pests that could be transmitted by the plants or plant products under consideration and against which no effective treatment can be applied or is not available for application
2	Partial embargoes	• Apply when a pests of quarantine importance to and an importing country is known to occur only in well defined area of the exporting country. • And an effective operating internal plant quarantine service exists that is able to contain pest or disease within this area.
3	Inspection & treatment at point of origin	• Inspection & treatment of given commodity when it originates from a country where pests/ diseases of quarantine significance to importing country is known to occurs.
4	Inspection & certification at point of origin	• Involves pre-shipment inspection by the importing country in assistance with exporting country and certification in accordance with quarantine requirement of importing country
5	Inspection at the point of entry	• Involves inspection of planting material instantly upon coming on at the prescribed port of entry and if required subject to treatment before the same disbursed
6	Utilization of post entry plant quarantine facilities	• Involvs growing of introduced plant propagating material under isolated and confined conditions

Plant quarantine in India

Sl.No	National legislations
1	Destructive Insects and Pests (DIP) Act of 1914
2	Plant Quarantine (Regulations of Import into India) Order 2003

3	Livestock Importation Act1898
4	The Environmental (Protection) Act 1986
5	Biological diversity Act 2002

- Destructive Insects and Pests (DIP) Act of 1914 of Central Government, which regulates the introduction of exotic diseases and pests into the country or their spread from one state or union territory to another. The Act also empowers the State Governments to frame suitable rules and issue notifications for inter-state movement of plant and plant material. Those rules are known as plant quarantine rules.
- The Agricultural Pests and Diseases Acts of various states, which suppress or prevent the spread of diseases and pests in areas within a state or union territory.

3. Domestic quarantine

- Under the DIP Act, the Directorate of Plant Protection, Quarantine and storage has the accountability to take the essential steps and regulate the inter-state movement of plants and plant material in order to prevent the further spread of destructive pest and diseases that have already entered the country.
- The solitary object of enforcing domestic quarantine is to prevent the spread of these diseases from infected to non-infected areas.
- Presently, domestic plant quarantine exists in following diseases and pests

Pest/Diseases	Host plant material	Restricted States	
		From	To
Wart (*Synchytrium endobioticum*)	Potato	Darjelling West Bengal	Any other state or place in India
Bunchy top (virus)of banana	Banana planting material	Assam, Kerala, Orissa, TamilNadu&West Bengal	Any other state or place in India &Uninon Territory
Mosaic (virus) of banana	Banana plants & planting material	Maharashtra &Gujarat	Any other state or place in India &Uninon Territory
Apple scab (*Venturia inaequalis*)	Apple planting materials	J&K and Himachal Pradesh	Any other states of India
Potato cyst nematodes (*Globodera rostochiensis* & *G pallida*)	Potato	Tamil Nadu	Any other state or place in India &Uninon Territory
Codling moth (*Carpocapsa pomenella*)	Apple and Walnut plants including fruits	Ladakh districts	Any other area of Jammu & Kashmir

Fluted Scale (*Icerya purchase*)	Many host plant	Mysore (Karnataka), Madras (Tamil Nadu) &Kerala	Any other state or place in India
Coffee berry borer (*Hypothena mushampei*)	Coffee seeds/plants/ powder	Nilgiri (TN), Kodagu (Karnataka) &Wynad (Kerala)	Any other states of India
San Jose Scale (*Aspidiotus perniciosus*)	Many host plant species	Punjab, UP, Madras (Tamil Nadu) &Kerala, WB, Assam, Orissa, HP, J&K	All other part of India

4. Pesticide Management Bill. 2020

The Pesticides Management Bill, 2020 is replacement of 50 years old Insecticide Act of 1968, approved by the Union Cabinet on 12 February 2020. It replaces the existing Insecticide Act, 1968, which Prakash Javadekar, the Minister for Information and Broadcasting, mentioned as "age-old and needs immediate rewriting". The aim of the Pesticides Management Bill, 2017 is to mainly

- Make in India.
- Made in India for the world.
- Ease of doing business.
- Aim should be " doubling of farmers income".
- Tremendous push for exports to make Indian production more competitive/ economical.
- Increase competition to reduce cost to the farmer.
- Fast track registrations to domestic R & D based manufacturing companies.
- Reduce dependence on imported, technical's& stop import of formulations.
- Register TECHNICAL 1st (as was happening for 40+ years , & do not register formulation directly).
- Control pests.
- Ensure availability of quality pesticides.
- Allow its use only after assessing its efficacy and safety.
- Minimize the contamination of agricultural commodities by pesticide residues.
- Create awareness among users regarding safe and judicious use of pesticides.
- To take necessary measures to continue, restrict or prohibit the use of pesticides with a view to prevent its risk on human beings, animals or environment.

PMB-2020 must encourage

1. Introduction of newer & better molecules.
2. Promote science-driven innovations.
3. Make India attractive investment destination.
4. Facilitate indigenous manufacture and exports to make India a global hub of supply.
5. Give farmers wide selection of pesticide molecules against pests, diseases, weeds.

Major areas of concern

1. Import of formulation is killing the Indian industry and does not provide level playing field.
2. Generic pesticide manufacturers are being treated as 'second grade citizens'.
3. Uncertainty about registration guidelines.
4. Too many arbitrary criteria to grant registration.
5. No time for grant /denial of registration.
6. Double whammy – licence to be revoked with conviction of an offence.
7. Arbitrariness of review process

9.6 Chemical Management

Farmers lose a considerable portion of income as their crops and produce are attacked by various insects, diseases and weeds leading to a significant reduction in crop productivity and lower actual yield than the attainable yield of crops. Yield losses caused by pests, pathogens, and weeds are responsible for 20–40% loss of global agricultural productivity. In India, 20-25% crop losses are reported due to pest attacks every year. As per Ministry of Agriculture, India is losing agricultural production worth INR 1.48 lakh crores annually due to damage from pests, weeds and plant diseases.

Recently, India fought a battle against desert locusts whose attack had wiped out lush green fields laden with crops like bajra, sorghum, maize, green gram, black gram, castor, wheat, cotton and vegetable crops spread over 50,000 hectares in Rajasthan, Gujarat, Madhya Pradesh, Uttar Pradesh, Punjab and Maharashtra. The use of insecticide Malathion helped very effectively in managing the situation. Plant protection chemicals are help in preventing rats, mice, flies and other insects from contaminating the food whilst in storage.

India lags in crop protection products usage

At present, only 25-30% cultivated area is covered by the crop protection umbrella. There is need for increased usage of crop protection products. The domestic market has enormous growth potential because of low pesticide use,which is among the lowest in the world. India's per hectare consumption of pesticide stands at 0.6kg/ha against the global average consumption of 3kg/ha. Per hectare consumption of pesticides in other countries like China at 4.57kg/ha,Japan 11.85 kg/ha and 13.06 kg/ ha. At present 1,175 molecules are available globally but about only 294 are registered in India. Only about 75 molecules and their combinations are being used to protect 140 million hectare of diverse Indian agricultural crops. In contrast, much smaller countries like Vietnam, Pakistan have over 500 registered molecules. USA, EU and Brazil have around 650/750 approved molecules for their farmers. Increase in pesticide consumption and bringing hither to untapped areas of cultivation under its umbrella will help to boost agriculture productivity and feed our increasing population.

Indian farmers need for greater range of newer molecules to fight the battle against pests, diseases, weeds and other attacks. The limited number of molecules lead to unintended consequences of spurious and fake products in the market, compounding the problem further. Therefore, Industry and government should work towards ensuring that the farmers are equipped with the best technologies to produce more from less in an environmentally sustainable manner.

Judicious use of pesticides

Poison-containing chemicals have been classified as medicine for plants and sold to farmers. The work of companies is not only the trade of chemicals, but also to create more and more profits. In the name of crop protection, the sale of poisonous chemicals increased. The pests developed higher resistance. In order to deal with them, the proportion of chemicals was further increased.For this purpose, they first create the disease and then treat the disease to make profits. The result is before us.

We have big data in support of crop protection chemicals. With the significant increase in production, the in debtedness of farmers is increasing too. Farmers are spending more and more on crop protection measures, but production not increased in the same proportion. Production has declined qualitatively, and also quantitatively – in terms of proportionate increase. One thing has happened for sure – the sale of crop safety chemicals has gone up multiple times.

Agriculture has a very important place in the making of AtmaNirbhar India. A joint consultation mechanism of the farmers, industrialists and the government is vital to check indiscriminate use of agro-chemicals for crop protection and also be mindful of their side effects. In the name of crop protection in modern farming, the use of poison containing chemicals was promoted in the name of scientific recommendations. For crop protection, the focus was solely on chemicals. The system of natural control of pests has been ignored.

Using pesticides at the right time, at economic threshold level (ETL), and minimizing their usage has a major role in crop protection. The use of pesticides for sustainable crop production was advocated by Nobel Peace Prize winner Dr NE Borlaug. Pesticides are a reliable source to keep pest population below ETL if used cautiously. The judicious usage of pesticides plays a key role in plant protection. Expert advice should be taken prior to deciding on a pesticide option. First, one has to confirm that the pest we want to manage is going to cross the ETL, which is the density of pest at which management measures should be applied.Farmers must quantify the damage caused by a particular pest after determining the ETL and apply pesticide accordingly. We educate farmers about the benefits of right usage of pesticides.

Need for equilibrium

We have to work with equilibrium at both the ecology and economy levels. The economy has to be developed on the basis of ecology. The side effect of chemicals is now becoming a problem. That is why there is a need to move forward responsibly on every aspect of agriculture in a planned manner. Farmers should develop farming methods by understanding the natural rules control and balance. Organic farming is a worthwhile option. The industry and the government must work together on biological molecular research instead of dependence on chemical molecules.

Crop protection products must be used discriminately, only after identification of the pest. All the work related to crop protection chemicals should be done in collaboration the Farmer Producer Organizations – not through the market.

The purpose of politics is to conserve and promote natural resources. Keeping this in mind, restrictions and control must be placed on the anti-nature elements of economic development. Such crimes must receive harsh punishment.

Life with nature is a necessity for human beings. Walking in opposition to the system of nature in the name of crop protection cannot be labeled as development. Most of the activities done solely with profit mentality are anti-nature. Life safety is more important than crop protection. The control mechanism for all kinds of insects, diseases and weeds is available in nature. We only need to decode and understand it. We welcome the decision of the government to ban harmful pesticides. All stakeholders must together to make India free of the use of poisonous chemicals.

Curbing counterfeit CPC

Crop Protection chemicals (CPC) play an important role in preventing crop losses both before and after harvesting.That's why the increasing incidence of counterfeit and illegally traded CPC in India is a serious issue. While legally registered CPC undergo rigorous testing under global and local regulations, illegal products are not tested for efficacy or impact on human health and environment. Counterfeit CPC may contain unknown, toxic impurities. The residues of these untested substances can be carried into harvested food and may compromise human and animal health. It can also pose health threats to farmers and farm workers through exposure during application. Manufacturing legal CPC involves significant investment and time for securing new registrations. Proliferation of illegal products results in loss of sales, patent and trademark infringement, erosion of data protection and damage to reputation. Illegal products also cause resistance in pests and manufacturers have to come up with newer technologies to replace old chemicals.

Government of India has a zero-tolerance position towards counterfeits and is committed to combating them as effectively as possible. They conduct regular awareness campaigns to educate farmers against the ill-effects of using counterfeit CPC.This is a part of our ongoing product stewardship strategy. Dealers and distributors can play an important role in discouraging the illegal sale and supply of counterfeit crop protection chemicals. Additionally, the enforcement department and the government's regulatory mechanism has to be more vigilant in curbing this menace.

Right policy and market environment

India needs to develop policies for improving farm-to-fork competitiveness of major crops. Innovations in modern crop protection and biotechnology have helped change the face of agriculture, offering farmers the benefit of efficiency, productivity, and sustainability. Innovation lies at the core of transforming food production. That's why India needs to accelerate introduction of new technologies in crop protection to match pace with other big agricultural nations. This means shortening product registration timelines and fast-tracking critical innovations for timely response to emerging threats like the Fall Army Worm impacting corn cultivation. In case of biotech regulatory reforms, they need to be introduced in conjunction with reforms for crop protection. This requires a holistic regulatory regime starting with breeding, crop protection to biotechnology to mitigate risk and improve yields significantly.For India to become a globally competitive manufacturing hub for crop protection products, we need enhanced data protection measures to safeguard the investment towards innovation and R&D of new products. With accelerated use of digital technologies and open knowledge platforms, there's a great opportunity to scale up our regulatory capacity including strong alliances for knowledge transfer with other leading countries. This again will be a strong foundation to accelerate regulatory reforms on a real time basis.

Robust regulatory system vital

The nation needs a robust regulatory system in place for vibrant crop protection. Improved regulations and implementation in relation to collecting and recording data on import, export, manufacture, formulation, quality and quantity of pesticides are essential for Indian agro produce to become globally competitive. As of now, we have inconsistent regulatory framework for control of pesticides, overlapping mandates for different agencies with pesticide management responsibilities and conflicting provisions regarding allowed pesticide uses. Joint reviews and inspection of fake and spurious pesticides is the need of the hour. Public confidence in pesticide regulatory processes and decisions needs to improve. In an un-starred question in the Lok Sabha on March 3, 2020, it was mentioned that in the last three years, out of 1,91,365 analyzed spurious samples, merely 2,584 are under prosecution stage. Further, there are over 250,000 registrations corresponding to only 292 registered pesticide molecules, i.e. close to 900 per molecule (process of issuing such registrations continues at an alarming pace). This has made way for non-serious players who have little regard for quality and standards. Getting a manufacturing license from the state-notified authority under the

Insecticide Act is not difficult either. By and large, it is given without checking for basic facilities, including quality control.

The result is an unmanageably large number of pesticide manufacturing units – currently over 1,400. Juxtaposed with poor enforcement of Insecticide Act and Insecticides Rules (1971), this has led to proliferation of spurious and substandard products and helps fly-bynight operators. The government must integrate all stakeholders in the value chain who function as the eyes and ears for inspecting the quality of pesticides. The government can enable joint review of pesticides to create a democratic environment for those who are working hard to make available the right quality ofpesticides.

Enabling policy needed

The Pesticide Management Bill 2020 is another opportunity to bring in a predictable progressive science-based legislation in place of the age old Insecticide Act of 1968. There is need for greater thrust on the manufacturing sector, which has been striving to get the best technologies to our farming community year after year. The R&D based crop sciences industry has been launching molecules that has over time led to reduced application rates. These were as high as1,000-3,000 grams of active ingredient per hectare in the case of molecules such as organophosphate and carbamate during the 1960s and 1970s. By the eighties, with the advent of cartap and synthetic pyrethroids, the dosages had come down to 50-500 grams per hectare. From the nineties to the early 2000s, there was further advancement giving way to triazoles and neonicotinoids, having dosages of 25- 200 grams per hectare. Since the mid- 2000s, the active ingredient application has fallen to less than 100 grams and in some cases of very low toxicity molecules– such as sulfonylureas and diamides –even as small as 4 grams per hectare.The pursuit towards greener chemistries continues and wishes encouragement to make our agriculture both economically viable through reduction of crop losses and more sustainable by reducing environmental load. It calls for creation of a policy environment that incentivizes a steady flow of the latest and safer products.

Fair review essential

If India today produces a record 291.95 million tonnes of food grain, it owes much to the introduction of CPP besides quality high yielding variety (HYV) seeds. Despite this, CPP come under intense scrutiny, reviews and criticism from NGOs and digital media. They have to prove their worth again and again. Admittedly, better products with the least environmental impact should be available to the farming communities. But one sees lack of enough scientific basis to the reviews and knee jerk reactions by way of bans, both at the Centre and State levels. A case in point is the recent proposal to ban 27 molecules by the Central Government. The scientific community has been generating scientific data on the efficacy as well as safety aspects of the various molecules and most importantly,the importance to the farming community in protecting their crops. The scientific community and farmers have been sending their feedback and representations to the government on the adverse consequences if the molecules are banned. Hopefully after due consideration the government will take an informed science based decision.

Role of Pesticides in IDM

Efficient, effective and safe disease management is not a case of "See a disease – spray a pesticide". It is a case of using all available techniques, all of which play a part in keeping diseases at levels below those which cause economic damage or loss – in other words, Integrated Disease Management. Pesticides more often than not are an integral component of an IDM programme.

The advantages of pesticides are that they provide an effective and quick reduction of diseases when numbers reach economically damaging levels, they can manage several diseases at the same time, and they are easy to use.

The disadvantages of pesticides are that they provide only a temporary solution, can be costly, involve a hazard in use and to the environment, can kill natural enemies of diseases, can cause disease resurgence, excessive use can result in disease resistance, and there is a potential risk to users and others. In IDM, therefore, pesticides are used only when diseases are causing, or will cause economic loss or damage. Crop monitoring and application thresholds are used to determine disease intensity and to time applications at the most vulnerable disease stage. If a pesticide is used, it ideally should be selective, of low persistence and of low toxicity.

Normally, pesticides are used when an examination of the crop shows that economically significant levels of the disease are present. However, there are situations where the preventative use of pesticides is desirable or essential such as seed dressings against soil-borne pathogens and early season disease vector control to limit virus infections of crop plants, and crop fungal diseases.

No attempt should ever be made to eradicate a disease with pesticides, as this is almost impossible to achieve. In addition, small numbers of diseases may be required to provide a food source for natural enemies, particularly parasites.

In addition, diseases may be present which are not normally a problem as their level are kept low by natural enemies. When a pesticide is applied, this control is removed as the natural enemies are killed, and the diseases can develop from secondary diseases to become major diseases. This is known as disease resurgence and is due to the pesticide killing the natural enemies of the diseases, as well as most, but not all, the diseases. The removal of the natural control allows the diseases to multiply to much higher levels than before. In addition, diseases may be present which are not normally a problem as their numbers are kept low by natural enemies. When a pesticide is applied, this control is removed as the natural enemies are killed, and the disease can develop from secondary disease to become major diseases. Choosing a product with restricted activity or that is specific to the disease, or spot application to areas of the crop with high disease level, can help avoid these problems.

Thresholds and Pest Scouting

- Thresholds are the disease level at which a pesticide application is needed in order to prevent economic loss or damage.

- They are set at the level where, if the disease level continues at that level or increases, then the value of the economic loss or damage would be greater than the cost of control.
- The economic threshold is calculated from a range of factors including the expected price for the produce, the expected yield, factors which may influence the yield and future disease attack (eg weather), and the anticipated cost of future control interventions.
- The economic threshold is thus dynamic, varying almost on a daily basis, and is thus difficult to apply in practice.

Spray threshold

- The pest level at which a pesticide treatment will give a return to the farmer in most seasons.
- Treatment thresholds can also vary during the season, based on such factors as crop growth stage, the damage or loss pests can cause at that stage, and the number of beneficial insects present.
- These variations are also derived from research trials, but the changes occur at pre-fixed intervals during the cropping season.
- With insect pest thresholds, a pest population is usually allowed to exist in the crop, as the cost of control would be greater than the value of the crop saved from loss or damage.

Disease scouting

- Disease scouting is the term given to monitoring a crop for levels of disease infestation, and natural enemies, and the growth stages of the pathogen.
- It is done on a regular basis, the intervals depending on the crop and the diseases of importance.
- Scouting also enables hot-spots of infestations to be identified and spot sprayed, rather than spraying the whole field.
- Scouting provides the information on whether disease levels are above or below the treatment threshold, and so if an intervention is needed or not, and information on whether previous control actions have been successful. Different crops and diseases have different disease scouting methods and techniques.
- The same crop and diseases may have different methods in different areas or countries. As a result, the treatment thresholds will also be different.
- Thresholds and pest scouting are one of the fundamental aspects of IPM and of the effective, efficient and economic use of pesticides.

Pesticide selection

- If it has been decided that a pesticide is essential, the correct pesticide must be used.

- A pesticide only controls a certain range of diseases, so one which is effective against the disease to be controlled must be selected.
- A pesticide should not be applied simply because it is a pesticide or is cheap – this is a waste of time and money if it is not effective against the diseases.
- If possible select a pesticide with a limited range of activity. Such a pesticide has the least effect on natural and reduces the risk of resistance in other pathogens.
- In the very early stages of an infestation, "mild" pesticides can be used, such as mineral oils against insects and mites, and micronised sulphur against mites and powdery mildew.
- If there is more than one suitable pesticide, select the one that poses the least risk to humans, animals and the environment under the conditions in which it will be used.
- A pesticide which is safer in these respects is not less effective in killing the target diseases.
- A fungicde of the same chemical group classification should not be used repeatedly in the same season against the same diseases or range of diseases. This increases the risk of pest resistance..
- Only pesticides from a reputable manufacturer or source should be used, and purchased in unopened or undamaged containers with a complete and undamaged label.
- Similarly, users (farmers) should only purchase pesticides from reputable pesticide retailers, in unopened and undamaged containers with a complete and undamaged label, and with a full crop season remaining before the expiry date.
- Counterfeit products are becoming more of a problem – these can be ineffective, as well as possibly dangerous to humans, animals and the environment, as well as being illegal.
- Users should be vigilant to avoid being sold counterfeit products, and be suspicious if offered products that are priced below the normal retail rate.

Pesticide dose rate

- The amount of pesticide applied per hectare is called pesticide dose rate. It have been evaluated by research and the manufacturers. These dose rates are given on the container label and should be followed when applying a pesticide.
- If too high a dose rate is applied, the excess is wasted. More pesticide is not more effective at controlling the diseases and the costs of control are increased. Also the risk of the pathogen developing resistance to the pesticide is increased.
- If too low a dose rate is applied, not all the diseases are controlled. Crop losses are not prevented, the use of the pesticide is not effective, and costs of control are increased.

- Dose rates are given on the container label either as the amount to apply per hectare, or as the amount to mix in so many litres of water at so many litres per hectare.

Causes of failure of pesticide applications

- The usual causes of poor results with an application of a genuine pesticide from a reputable source are:
- Incorrect pesticide for the diseases.
- Incorrect timing of the application.
- Incorrect dose rate.
- Incorrect application.
- Substandard pesticide .
- Pathogen resistance to the pesticide.
- Little absorption or movement of the pesticide within the plant.

Pesticide resistance in pathogen

Pesticide resistance is the inherited ability to tolerate the toxic effects of a pesticide.

- Every pathogen population contains a small proportion of individuals with this inherited ability.
- When a pesticide is applied, susceptible individuals are killed while the resistant individuals survive.
- The proportion of resistant individuals in the population is thus increased.
- This effect occurs each time a pesticide is applied, with the proportion of resistant individuals increasing every time.
- As the proportion of resistant individuals increases, the normal dose of pesticide is not enough for effective control, and higher doses or more frequent applications are required.
- Eventually the proportion of resistant individuals in the population is so large that it is impossible to control the pathogen with the pesticide.

Factors encourage development of resistance in pathogen

Factors which encourage the development of resistance in pathogen population are:

- Using too high a dose of the pesticide. A greater proportion of the susceptible individuals are killed, so resistant individuals are more likely to mate or spread infective inoculum.

- Using the same pesticide, or pesticides from the same chemical group, too frequently in the same season. The pathogens are continually exposed to the pesticide, which eliminates the susceptible individuals much more rapidly.
- Using a pesticide with a long persistence. The pathogens are continually exposed to the pesticide, which eliminates the susceptible individuals much more rapidly.
- The proportion of resistant individuals in the population before the pesticide is used. The higher the proportion to begin with, the faster resistance will develop.
- Exposure of a greater proportion of the pathogen population to the pesticide, such as with area-wide treatments.
- Resistance can build up more quickly with pathogen that multiply rapidly.

Factors minimise the development of resistance

Factors which minimise the development of resistance in a pathogen population are:

- Applying pesticides only when necessary.
- Using pesticides from different groups during the season.
- Using the correct pesticide dose rate.
- Applying the pesticide effectively.
- Using less persistent pesticides.
- A long pathogen disease cycle.
- Following IDM principles.

Combination fungicides

Combination fungicides is a formulation of two or more active ingredients. The combined fungicides broaden the spectrum of activity and increase the potency of each treatment. Increased potency further reduces pathogen populations, leading to a longer duration of control. It also reduces the risk of resistance to individual fungicides or fungicide classes and can lessen stress-induced mutation among survivors. Concert (propiconazole + chlorothalonil, Syngenta), Honor (pyraclostrobin + boscalid, BASF) and Instrata (propiconazole + chlorothalonil + fludioxonil, Syngenta) were among the earliest introduced into markets.

The research says ...

- Combination fungicide products provide optimized formulations of two or more active ingredients and the convenience of one product.
- Combination products reach more pathogens with a single application and will result in a greater reduction in pathogen populations.
- Combining fungicides can limit exposure to each active ingredient, reducing selection for pathogen strains with resistance to each individual fungicide.

Advantages of combining fungicides for disease control

1. **Reaching more pathogens:** One of the disease-control advantages of combining fungicides into a single formulation is to broaden the spectrum of activity of the treatment — that is, to reach more target pathogens with a single application.
2. **Increasing potency:** A second advantage is to increase the potency of the treatment — a benefit that has both direct and indirect influence on disease control. From a direct perspective, two active ingredients are more likely to kill the target pathogen than either individually.
3. **Fungicide resistance management:** Indirect benefits of increasing the potency of the treatment involve fungicide resistance management. The rise of resistance is driven by two factors — selection pressure and mutation. Combining fungicides can limit exposure to each active ingredient, thereby reducing selection pressure for pathogen strains with resistance to each individual fungicide.

Approved formulation of combination fungicides in India

SI.No.	Combination Product	Company
1.	Ametoctradin 27% + Dimethomorph 20.27 % SC	BASF India Ltd. Mumbai
2.	Azoxystrobin 4.8% w/w+Chlorothalonil 40.0 % w/w SC	M/s SyngentaIndia Ltd.
3.	Azoxystrobin 18.2% + Cyproconazole 7.3% w/w SC	M/s SyngentaIndia Ltd.
4.	Azoxystrobin 8.3% + Mancozeb 66.7 % WG	M/s United Phosphorus Ltd.,
5.	Azoxystrobin 1 1.5 % + Mancozeb 30.0 % WG	M/s Crystal Crop Protection Pvt. Ltd., Delhi
6.	Azoxystrobin 16.7 % + Tricyclazole 33.3 % SC	M/s Crystal Crop Protection Pvt. Ltd., Delhi
7.	Azoxystrobin 11.0 % + Tebuconazole 18.3% SC	M/s GSP Crop Science Pvt. Ltd., Ahmedabad
8.	Azoxystrobin 12.5% + Tebuconazole 12.5% SC	M/s Excel Crop Care Ltd. Mumbai
9.	Azoxystrob in 7.1 % + Propiconazole 11.9 % SE	M/s Adama Makhteshim Ltd
10.	Benalaxyl-M 4.0 % + Mancozeb 65.0 % WP	M/s Isagro (Asia) Agrochemical Pvt. Ltd.
11.	Benalaxyl 18.0 % + Mancozeb 65 % WP	M/s FMC India Ltd.
12.	Boscalid 25.2 + Pyraclostrobin 12.8 % WG	M/s BASF India Ltd., Mumbai
13.	Captan 70 % + Hexaconazole 5 % WP	

SI.No.	Combination Product	Company
14.	Carbendazim 12 % + Mancozeb 63 % WP	M/s United Phosphorus Ltd., Mumbai.
15.	Carbendazim 12 % + Mancozeb 63 % WS	M/s United Phosphorus Ltd., Mumbai
16.	Carbendazim 1.92 % + Mancozeb 10.08 % GR	M/s United Phosphorus Ltd., Mumbai
17.	Carbendazim 25 % + Mancozeb 50 % WS	M/s Indofil Industries Ltd.
18.	Carbendazim 25 % Flusilazole 12.5 % SE	M/s Dhanuka Agritech Ltd.
19.	Carboxin17.5%+Thiram17.5%FF	M/s Chemchura Chemical Pvt. Ltd.
20.	Carboxin 37.5 % + Thiram 37.5 % WS	M/s Crompton Specialaties Asia Pacific.
21.	Carfentrazone Ethyl 20 % + Sulfosulfuron 25 % WG	M/s FMC India Pvt. Ltd., Bangalore
22.	Cartaphydrochloride 4% + Fipronil 0.5 % w/w CG	M/s Willo Wood Chemicals Pvt. Ltd.
23.	Copper Sulphate 47.15% + Mancozeb 30% WDG	M/s UPL Ltd. Mumbai
24.	Cymoxanil 8% + Mancozeb 64%WP	
25.	Dimethomorph 12% + Pyraclostrobin 6.7 % WG	M/s BASF India Pvt. Ltd., Mumbai
26.	Famoxadone 16.6 % + Cymoxanil 22.1 % SC	M/s El Dupont India Pvt. Ltd, Gurgaon
27.	Fenamidone 10 % + Mancozeb 50 % WDG (FI)	M/s Bayer Crop Science Ltd
28.	Fenamidone 4.44 % + Fosetyl-AI 66.66 % WDG (FI)	M/s Bayer Crop Science Ltd
29.	Fluocoplide 4.44 % + Fosetyl-AI 66.66 % WDG (FI)	M/s Bayer Crop Science Ltd
30.	Fluopicolide 5.56 % w/w + Propamocarbhydrochloride 55.6 % w/w SC	M/s Bayer Crop Science Ltd
31.	Fluopyram 17.7% + Tebuconazole 17.7% SC	M/s Bayer Crop Science Ltd., Mumbai
32.	Fluxapyroxad 250 g/l + Pyraclostrobin 250 g/l SC (FI)	M/s BASF India Ltd., Mumbai
33.	Fluxapyroxad 167 g/L + Pyraclostrobin 333g/lSC (FI)	M/s BASF India Ltd.,Mumbai
34.	Fluxapyroxad 62.5g/l + epoxiconazole 62.5g/l EC	M/s BASF India Ltd., Mumbai
35.	Hexaconazole 4% + Carbendazim 16 % w/w SC	M/s Insecticide India Ltd.
36.	Hexaconazole 5% + Validamycin 2.5 % SC	M/s Willowoodchem.Pvt Ltd.
37.	Hexaconazole 4% + Zineb 68 % WP	M/s Indofil Industries Ltd.

SI.No.	Combination Product	Company
38.	Improvalicarb 5.5% + Propineb 61.25 % WP	M/s Bayer Crop Science Ltd
39.	lprodion 25 % + Carbendazim 25 % WP	M/s Aventis Cropscience Ltd., Mumbai
40.	Kasugamycin 5 % + Copper Oxychloride 45 % WP	M/s. Dhanuka Agritech Ltd.
41.	Mancozeb 40 % + Azoxytrobin 7.0 %w/ WOS	M/s Coromandel International Ltd., Telangana
42.	Mandipropamid 5.0 % w/w + Mancozeb 60.0 % w/w WG	M/s Syngenta India Limited
43.	Metalaxyl-M3.3 % + Chlorothalonil 33.1 % SC	M/s Syngenta India Ltd.,
44.	Metalaxyl- M 8 % + Mancozeb 64 % WP	M/s Syngenta India Ltd, Pune
45.	Metalaxyl- M 4% + Mancozeb 64 % WP	M/s Syngenta India Ltd.
46.	Metiram 55 % + Pyraclostrobin 5% WG (Fl)	M/s BASF India Ltd.
47.	Metiram 44 % + Dimethomorph 9% w/w WG (Fl)	M/s BASF India Ltd.
48.	Penflufen13.28 % w/w + Trifloxystrobin 13.28 w/w FS	M/s Bayer Cpyriproamrop Science Ltd
49.	Picoxystrobin 6.78 % + Tricyclazole 20.33 % SC	M/s E.I. Dupont India Private Ltd,
50.	Picoxystrobin 7.05 % + Propiconazole1 1.71 % SC	M/s E.I. Dupont India Private Ltd,
51.	Propiconazole1 0.7% + Tricyclazole 34.2 % SE	M/s Syngenta India Ltd, Pune
52.	Propiconazole1 3.9% + Difenoconazole 13.9% EC	M/s Syngenta India Ltd.
53.	Propineb 54.2 % + Tricyclazole1 5.0 % WP	M/s Coromandel International Ltd., Telangana
54.	Pyroclostrobin 133g/I + Epoxiconazole 50g/I (w/v) SE (FI}	M/s BASF India Ltd.
55.	Pyrithiobac Sodium 6 % + Quizalofop Ethy 14 % w/wEC	M/s Godrej Agrovet Ltd., Mumbai
56.	Quizalofopethy 10% EC + Chlorimuronethyl 25 % WP + Surfactant (0.2}	M/s. Dhanuka Agritech Ltd., New Delhi
57.	Quizalofopethy 14% + Pyrithiobacsodium 6.0 % w/wEC	M/s Godrej Agrovet Ltd., Mumbai
58.	Streptomycin + Tetracycline {90+10}	M/s Hindustan Antibiotics Ltd., Mumbai
59.	Tebuconazole 6.7% + Captan 26.9 % w/w SC	M/s. ADAMA India Pvt. Ltd.,
60.	Tebuconazole10 % + Sulphur 65% WG	M/s Excel Crop Care Ltd., Mumbai
61.	Tebuconazole 50 % + Trifloxystrobin 25% WG **(Fl)**	M/s Bayer Crop Science Ltd., Mumbai

SI.No.	Combination Product	Company
62.	Thiophanate Methyl 450 g/L + Pyroclostrobin 5g/LFS **(FI)**	M/s. BASF India Ltd.
63.	Triafamone 20 % w/w + Ethoxysulfuron10 % WG % w/w, SC 390 RC	M/s Bayer Crop Science Ltd., Mumbai
64.	Tricyclazole 45 % + Hexaconazole 10 % WG	M/s Indofil Industries Ltd.
65.	Tricyclazole 18.0 w/w + Tebuconazole 14.4 % w/w SC	M/s Dow Agroscience India Pvt. Ltd., Mumbai
66.	Tricyclazole18 % + Mancozeb 62% WP	M/s Indofil Industries Ltd.
D. INSECTICIDE+FUNGICIDE		
1.	Flubendiamide 3.5% + Hexaconzole 5 % WG	M/s Rallis India Ltd.,
2.	Imidacloprid 18.5 % + Hexaconzole 1.5 % FS	M/s Rallis India Ltd.,

Drone usage in Agrochemical Spraying

Drones have proven to be among the most promising technologies emerging from the fourth Industrial Revolution. Drone usage in agrochemical spraying can have a major impact on Indian farms and needs government support for enabling supportive policy framework.

The main benefits of drones in spraying of agrochemicals are the following:

1. Increased efficiency and precision of agrochemical application. This leads to improved pest management and crop productivity, eliminates or reduces wastage of crop protection products (CPP).
2. Significant reduction in risk of operator exposure during spray operations.Field capacity of drone-assisted spraying is over 20 times higher compared to manual spraying.
3. Lower water consumption.
4. Development of certified applicators, including community spraying professionals providing application services, thereby creating new skilled employment and entrepreneurship potential in rural India.
5. Certain special field conditions (such as deserts or hilly terrains) and crop growth stages are more suitable for spraying through drones.
6. Mitigate emerging trends in labour shortage.

Admittedly, there are risks involved in any new technology. For drones, these are flight risks, risks to the operator, by stander, the crop and also the environment. It is important to study how other countries are using pragmatic regulations for mitigating these risks.

Indian Scenario

In recent years, use of drone in agriculture has gained attention. Drones have been used to fight highly mobile invasive pests such as Fall Armyworm (FAW) and desert locusts efficiently and effectively;prevent them from becoming endemic while maintaining high agricultural productivity. Recently Government of India, as a special case has recommended usage of drones for spraying operations to control the locust as band application to save the crops. Some state governments have issued e-tenders for inclusion of drones in aerial pesticide applications. Ministry of agriculture has come up with broad specification for drones that can fly at night and stay airborne fornight duty in locust control, making India the first country to do so. There is opportunity to extend it to other pests and areas of application through robust and pragmatic science-based policy framework. Progress has been made on the subject in setting guidelines for "Krishi drones" as envisioned in the ICAR expert committee appointed by the Ministry of Agriculture.

Agrochemical traceability

1. Most companies still rely on paper-based tracking systems which are time-consuming, manual and inefficient.
2. Good traceability enables producers, distributors and consumers to track the movement of goods.
3. Traceability innovation means.
    - To have the tools at our disposal for a fully harmonized, end-to-end supply chain solution.
    - It can track a formulated product from conceptualization to the field.

Track and Trace Technology

This can help stakeholders with the following operations

- Demand forecasting.
- Anti-counterfeiting measures.
- Sustainable purchasing.
- Inventory management.
- Recall management.
- Consumer engagement tools.
- Loyalty programs.
- Real-time supply chain visibility.
- Decision-making tools with data analysis.

Traceability will help answer the following questions:

- How can one assure customers that my product is safe?
- How can one prove that my ingredients are sustainably sourced?

- How can our customers be sure that my product is not counterfeit?

Benefits

- Increased transparency of products.
- Transactional efficiency.
- Reduced costs.
- Fewer staff redundancies.
- Collaborative potential for enhancing the workflows.
- Expanded sales of highvalue products.
- Larger net revenues for all stakeholders.

10

Spurious Pesticides

Introduction

Pesticides have a direct impact on agricultural economy and food security. The presence of spurious, fake, illegal or duplicate pesticides in the market result in losses of yield and farmers' income. Over 30% of plant protection chemicals sold in India are not registered, fake, sub-standard, misbranded, counterfeit, unapproved and illegitimate pesticides, bio pesticides and bio-stimulants. They are developed by passing regulations and field trials. These spurious products are sold with the strong nexus of manufacturers, retailers and the local administration. The magnitude of the problem can be assessed from the fact that the market size of spurious pesticides was worth Rs 3,200 crore of total pesticides market of Rs 16,900 crore in 2002, as per Tata Strategic Management Group (TSMG) and FICCI report. The report estimates the proportion of counterfeit pesticides as high as 40% in 2019. The use of such pesticides is growing at about 20% every year. Uttar Pradesh, Madhya Pradesh, Maharashtra, Andhra Pradesh, Karnataka, Haryana and West Bengal are among the worst-affected states. As per research done by Indian Institute of Public Administration with the help of Ministry of Consumer Affairs, 58% of agri inputs are fake in rural India. Indian farmers are mostly guided by retailers who follow unethical and illegal practices. They lure the farmers in an illusion of cost-effective solutions to purchase non genuine plant protection chemicals. Most farmers purchase spurious pesticides thinking that they are purchasing the original product.

Spurious pesticides

A pesticide shall be deemed to be spurious if

- An imitation of, or is sold under the name of, another pesticide.
- Shows active ingredient higher or lower than the limits prescribed on test or analysis.
- Not registered or licensed in the manner required by or under the Act.
- The container bears the name of the person or company purporting to be the manufacturer of the pesticide, which is either fictitious or counterfeit
- The chemical composition is not adhered to as approved by the Registration Committee.
- It has outlived its shelf-life, as evident by the date of manufacture and the date of expiry as printed on its label.

- It is found to be imported, manufactured, stocked, distributed, transported, sold despite its import, manufacture, use or sale is prohibited.

Implication of spurious pesticides

Spurious pesticides have a low or no impact on pests as compared to genuine pesticides and hence, a lower yield than expected is obtained by the farmer.

1. Implications on end users

- Pose danger to the farmer's health.
- Farmer would suffer economically due to crop loss..
- Yield of the farm can decrease.
- Usage of spurious pesticides destroys the fields and harvests forever as no antidotes available for farms.
- Lead to poverty and social unrest in the rural sector.

2. Implications on industry

- Due to the presence of "look alike" and "exact copies", the farmer loses trust in honest companies.
- Industry faces loss of sales, patent & trademark infringement, damage to reputation and problems in stewardship activities.
- Cause resistance in pests and therefore, the manufacturers have to come up with a newer technology to replace the older product.
- Many smaller indigenous companies may lead to loss of exports ultimately the image of Indian pesticide exports gets tarnished in outside countries.

3. Implications on government

- Poses a risk to present production of food grains, fruits and vegetables ultimately financial loss to the farmers.
- Rejection of exports.
- Loses its share in the tax coming from the pesticide market.
- Impact the government's image at international platforms.

4. Implications on Public

- Serious health problems for the society.
- Jeopardize the food security of the nation.
- Create a negative impression in the minds of the citizens about the working of the government machinery.
- Contamination of soil and ground water.

5. Implications on environment

- Reduces the soil fertility.
- Degrade the ground water reserves and also impact some useful pests in the long run.
- Cause resistance in pests which has environmental implications and economic implications.
- Left residues in soil that could be harmful to succeeding crops and can affect natural habitats of flora and fauna.

Key drivers of spurious pesticides

There exists a variety of reasons that leads to the proliferation of the spurious pesticides in the market. Some of these drivers are discussed below:

- The existing Insecticide Act 1968 is not being implemented by the Law Enforcing Machinery in its true spirit.
- The pesticide inspector visits the shops in the allotted area only once a month even in the peak season. It is often noticed that the schedule of his visits are already known to the distributers and retailers and the counterfeiters are able to hide their spurious pesticides. In addition, most distributers and retailers convince the pesticide inspector with unethical means to draw samples only from products of reputed companies.
- Long and burdensome registration process for fresh registration is a major restraint to the market and due to this reason many counterfeiters in high.
- Margin on spurious pesticides is very high (as much as 25-30%) as compared to 3%-5% in branded products.
- Price of the spurious pesticides may be up to 30-40% lower than the authentic brand which attracts farmers to use these spurious pesticides.
- There are multiple bio products being sold in the market. These products do not have any registration certificate number issued by CIB & RC. These products are laced with unknown chemicals and are totally untested for any kind of health, environmental or performance parameters.
- Some distributers and retailers mix packets of original branded pesticide with the exact copies" of the packaging and make a bigger carton. Hence, it becomes extremely difficult for the customer to differentiate between authentic and illegal product.
- Illegal imports constitute 30% of spurious pesticides in India. Either the total formulation or active ingredient is imported from organized crime rackets in outside countries to organized crimes in the country.
- If the companies are issued show-cause notices and their quality control heads are asked to explain the deficiencies in their products, they adopt "delaying tactics" by asking for a re-test from the Central Laboratory. In majority of cases,

the samples pass the re-test. This testing information is not posted publically and therefore access to information is limited.

- There exists a lack of education and awareness at the farmer level.

Technical grades most affected by spurious pesticides in India

Insecticides are the most affected genre of pesticide. Insecticide constitute ~70% of non-genuine / illegal pesticides market followed by fungicides which constitute ~20% of the market in India. Moreover, Copper Oxychloride, Buprofenzin, Fibronil, Imidacloprid, Flubendiamide, Emamectin Benzoate are are some of the active ingredients where percentage of non-genuine / illegal pesticides is highest.

Suggestions

1. Government level

- Government should decrease import duty from 10% to either 0 or 5% so newer molecules to be imported in India. They can serve the need of dealing with newer varieties of pests and other insects which develop resistance to older varieties of pesticides.
- Custom officers should be trained to identify fake products with the help of technology.
- Appoint nodal officers who will verify the licenses of distributors and retailers, seize samples and inspect the manufacturing sites and make this information public.
- List the prescribed pesticides, target pests, usage on crops and dosage on a portal.
- Make it mandatory for the pesticide inspectors to report back their on field findings about whether the pesticide is genuine or non-genuine.
- Reward a person who gives correct information about an illegal activity.
- Mandate a minimum educational requirement to qualify as pesticide retailer.
- Empower the village Panchayat to identify genuine retailers & take action against people dealing in spurious pesticides.
- Adoption of digital communication for faster connect with our farming community.
- Stringent action must be taken against those involved in supplying spurious or illegal pesticides and bio-pesticides/bioproducts laced with pesticides.

2. Farmers level

- Farmer community at village level should identify authorized retailers and encourage farmers to ask for a receipt after each purchase.
- Farmers should continue to attend awareness trainings organized by Government and the agro chemical companies.

- Farmers should utilize customer care telephone number written on the packaging to validate the authenticity of the product.
- Extension officials should distribute written material/leaflets containing information / warning against spurious pesticides.

3. Industry level

- Publicize success stories of farmers.
- Make distributors realize the importance of use of branded genuine products for farmers.
- Invest in farmer education programs for identifying authentic products and educate ill effects of spurious pesticides.
- Provide special helpline telephone numbers to resolve farmer's queries.

Challenges

- Difficult to reach farmers due to lack of proper communication with farmers.
- Multiplicity of languages and dialects, reluctance in adopting new technologies and new products.
- Farmers fear crop loss and are sceptical of new products. This makes popularisation of new genuine pesticides difficult amongst farmers.
- Nexus between retailers and distributors. They are taking advantage of the situation by pushing spurious products.
- Lack of adequate technical expertise also makes product understanding difficult for farmers.
- Reluctance of scientific community, leaders and stakeholders in agriculture to raise this issue in the interest of the farming community and prosperity of the nation.

11

Ecological Disease Management

In order for a plant to become diseased, three conditions must be present: (1) a pathogen, (2) a favorable environment and (3) a susceptible host. All the strategies we use to manage plant diseases work to remove or limit one of these factors, thus breaking the plant disease triangle. The key to sustainable plant disease management is to establish an agro- ecological system that is favorable to plant growth and development at the population level and adverse to pathogen evolution and epidemic development based on interactions among plants, pathogens, vectors and environment. The core of ecological plant disease management is to manipulate the environments of host-pathogen interactions in the favor of host through the balanced application of RAER (resistance, avoidance, elimination and remedy) strategy.

A. Host resistance

- Most convenient and effective approach of plant disease management.
- It can be quantitative or qualitative, local or systemic or induced or constitutive.
- Quantitative(minor gene) resistance is
  - Less effective.
  - Reduce disease epidemics rather than preventing infection.
  - More durable due to the lower selection pressure it places on pathogens.
- Qualitative (or major gene) resistance is
  - Highly effective.
  - Lose their effectiveness only a few years after commercial release, particularly when they are used in large-scale monocultures.
  - It is due to elevated evolution of plant pathogens under modern agricultural practices.
- Increasing host heterogeneity through intercropping or mixing crop varieties with different genetic and physiological properties such as type of resistance (qualitative versus quantitative) has been proved to be one of the most effective ecological approaches to manage plant diseases.
- This approach not only reduces disease epidemics, increases nutrition efficiency, productivity and yield stability in short term but also improves soil fertility and slows down pathogen evolution .

- In addition to mixture or intercropping technologies, other approaches in resistance gene deployment, such as R gene rotation and pyramiding, can also be used to assist in the ecological management of plant diseases

B. Avoidance & Elimination

a.Manage the Pathogen

1.Exclusion

- Keep the pathogens out.
- Make sure that your seeds and transplants are free of pathogens.
- The epidemic of late blight in Irish in 1845 was partially the result of the widespread distribution of the pathogen on infected seeds.
- Consider growing your own transplants/seeds; otherwise, inspect them carefully before you bring them to the farm.
- Saving seed can easily carry over pathogens from the previous year. Only save seed from healthy plants to reduce this risk.
- Although pathogens may occasionally be introduced from a commercial seed source, generally they are the most reliable source .
- Keep your equipment and stakes clean and sanitized. You don't want to be the grower who has bacterial spot in your peppers every year because you reuse your stakes without sanitizing them.
- Sodium hypochlorite at 0.5 percent is effective and must be followed by rinsing and proper disposal of solution. Prior to sanitizing, remove visible organic debris from the stakes and/or equipment.
- Any materials to be used on certified farms must be cleared with your certifier before use to prevent mishaps that could result in losing certification.

2. Eradicate or reduce the inoculum

- Crop rotation between plant families can help to keep the levels of disease down.
- Rotating to remediate a disease problem can be challenging, especially if the pathogen is long-lived in the soil and/or has a wide host range.
- Rotating between unrelated crops such as beans to sweet corn, lettuce to cucurbits, and cucurbits to crucifers can help avoid the buildup of soilborne pathogens .
- A good rule of thumb is that no crop family should return to the same field or bed for a minimum of three years to avoid soilborne disease buildup.
- Beware, some pathogens create special structures that allow them to survive in the field for much longer.

- Many pathogens can survive on debris over the winter. Tilling in plant residue at the end of the season allows soil microorganisms to break the material down, leaving potential pathogens without a host.

3. Antagonistic plants

- Certain plants, such as mustards and sudangrass, can kill plant pathogens that live in the soil.
- They contain a chemical and an enzyme in their plant tissue, specifically their cell wall.
- When we mow the plant and crush the tissue, the enzyme reacts with the chemical to create a toxic gas—the same as a fumigant. If you quickly incorporate this crushed plant material into the soil after mowing, the volatilized chemical can kill plant pathogens, nematodes, and weed seeds.
- Farmers in Northampton County tried this method to control plant-parasitic nematodes.
- However, the process can be tricky. We need to make sure we have the right varieties, enough moisture, adequate fertility, and good timing to get the result we want.

4. Hot water treatments

- If seed is affected by plant pathogens, use a hot water bath that will both surface disinfect as well as kill pathogens within the seed.
- For example, hot water treatment for eggplant submerses seeds in 122°F water for 25 minutes.
- Be careful to find out the correct temperature and length of time for the treatment. Too cold will not work and too hot will kill the seed .

5. Crop rotation affects pathogen persistence

- Clubroot, caused by *Plasmodiophora brassica*, can be a significant problem in brassica crops. The pathogen can survive in the soil for over seven years, even in the absence of mustard family crops or weeds.
- But clubroot tends to decline more quickly when tomato, cucumber, snap bean, and buckwheat are grown.
- Clubroot was effectively controlled by growing aromatic herbs including peppermint, garden thyme, and summer savory for two to three consecutive years . For some brassica crops, resistant varieties are also an option.

b. Create an unfavorable environment

1. Keep leaves dry

- Most fungi and bacteria that kill plants require wet environments from dew, rain, or irrigation to infect and cause disease.

- If we want to keep them from reproducing, don't give them the environment they like.
- Good air circulation and drip irrigation help keep the leaves dry and the diseases out.
- For example, gray mold in tomatoes is generally not a problem in the field. But, when you pack tomatoes in a high tunnel with little air circulation, it becomes common, especially within the lower portion of the plant.

2. Maintain high-quality soil

- Balanced fertility, good drainage, and good soil tilth will all help in promoting a diverse range of soil microorganisms.
- Diverse microbial communities generally compete with plant-pathogenic organisms in the soil and help keep your plants healthier.
- Plants that are not stressed are less susceptible to disease.

3. Manage weeds

- Many weeds are also hosts for diseases.
- When your crop is surrounded by weeds, the atmosphere tends to be moist, favoring infection.

C. Remedy

- Pesticides application to kill the pathogen or insect vectors is mandatory part of plant disease management when other management approaches cannot achieve the required level of disease reduction and epidemic amelioration .
- Judicious use of pesticides in an IDM system is not to eradicate the disease completely but to manage it below ecological and economical thresholds.
- Pesticides should be used in combination with disease forecasts and knowledge of the pathogen population genetic structure to determine the best time and frequency of application and to choose the type and utilization dosage of the pesticides.
- It helps in increasing the efficiency of application and reduce negative impacts of fungicides on the environment.
- Success could also be achieved by other approaches than pesticides like application of biological control and botanicals.
- During pesticide application, factors such as action modes and pathogen resistance should be considered .
- Combining pesticides with other biotic and abiotic approaches such as biological agents, soil pH adjustment and UV irradiation has proved to be very effective in long-term management of tomato and lettuce root rot

Ecological engineering for disease management

Of late, ecological engineering for disease management has emerged as a model of disease management approaches that rely on the use of cultural techniques to effect habitat manipulation and to enhance biological control. The cultural practices are rely on ecological knowledge than on high technology approaches like pesticides and genetic engineering crops.

Ecological engineering for disease management–Above ground

- Growing of compatible cash crops or flowering plants along the field border by arranging shorter plants towards main crops and taller plants towards the border to attract natural enemies and to avoid immigrating pathogen population.
- Do not uproot weed plants which are growing naturally like Ageratum sp., Alternanthera species, *Tridex procumbens* which act as nectar source for natural enemies.
- Growing flowering plants on the internal bunds inside the field.
- Broad spectrum synthetic chemical pesticides should not be applied when the P: D ratio is favorable. The plant compensation ability should also be considered before applying chemical pesticides.

Ecological engineering for disease management – Below ground

- Keep soils covered with living vegetation or crop residue throughout the year.
- Crop rotations with leguminous crop which enhance nitrogen content.
- Add organic matter in the form of farm yard manure, compost, vermicompost, crop residue which enhance below ground diversity.
- Reduce tillage intensity so that hibernating natural enemies can be conserved.
- Apply balanced dose of nutrients using biofertilizers to the soil.
- Apply mycorrhiza and plant growth promoting rhizobacteria (PGPR)
- Apply *Trichoderma viride/harzianum* and *Pseudomonas fluorescens* as seed /seedling, nursery treatment and soil application to reduce disease level and promote growth of the crop

12

Introduction to Conventional (Synthetic) Pesticides for Disease Management

Introduction

Of late, there has been a growing trend for individuals and companies to **"Go Green"** or be more environmentally friendly. There has also been a opinion that natural and organic products are healthier or safer. The pest control industry has responded to these changes in our culture and business markets with innovations in products, materials, and methods. Requests for "organic" based services have grown to a point where most pest control providers offer services that use only natural pesticides. However, words like, organic, natural and green have started to become cliché. So what does it really mean in regards to pesticides? For the sake of clarity, natural pesticides refer to products that are derived strictly from sources in nature with little to no chemical alteration. Synthetic pesticides are products that are produced from chemical alteration.

Know the difference

Synthetic (Conventional) pesticides

- Synthetic pesticides are often referred to as conventional pesticides.
- A substance that is formulated by a chemical process or by a process that chemically changes a substance extracted from naturally occurring plant, animal, or mineral sources.
- Some synthetically produced pesticides meet the criteria for use in organic agriculture. For example, copper sulfate and paracetic acid can be used for plant disease management.

Organic (Natural) pesticides

- **Organic pesticides** are generally considered to be pesticides derived from naturally occurring sources such as minerals, plants, or animals.
- These naturally occuring chemicals are broken down relatively quickly by weathering or soil microbes.
- Examples of organic pesticides include diatomaceous earth (fossilized water microbes), neem oil (a tree oil extract), or pyrethrins (an extract from chrysanthemums).

Origin does not dictate toxicity

- Regardless of whether a pesticide is organic or synthetic, it can still be dangerously toxic in certain doses.
- Organic pesticides are typically viewed as safer alternatives to synthetic pesticides, this is not always the case.
- It is essential that you read the label to determine the toxicity of each pesticide you use.
- Follow all label directions to protect yourself and the environment.
- Some organic pesticides carry the highest toxicity signal word, DANGER. For example, lime-sulfur solution, an effective fungicide, carries the DANGER signal word.
- This organic pesticide should be used with extreme caution.
- Conversely, simply because a pesticide is synthetic does not mean it is highly toxic. For example, the Virginia Cooperative Extension 2 fungicide Armada 50 WDG, carries a CAUTION label on the product. The point to remember is that organic does not mean "safe," just as synthetic does not mean "dangerous."
- Read the label to determine the hazards of each product you use.
- Choose the pesticide that best meets your needs.

What is better: Natural or Synthetic pesticides?

It can be hard to define what is better when you are choosing pesticides. When choosing a pesticide, you have to ask yourself what better looks like for you. For example, you may need to go with natural pesticides if you are planning to cultivate an organic garden.If you need immediate relief from pesticides, a fast-acting synthetic formula might be better for you. But in recent years, so-called natural, or "organic", pesticides have been growing in popularity. This has caused a boom in the natural pesticide market.

Advantages and disadvantages of natural pesticides

Advantages of using natural pesticides

1) Friendly to the environment.
2) Healthier.
3) Work better over the long run.
4) Better for the quality of your soil.
5) Going green.

Disadvantages of using natural pesticides

1) May be more costly than synthetic ones.
2) Some products may be less effective.

3) Delay action.
4) Require more knowledge to properly use them
5) Not as many companies offer natural chemicals yet.

Advantages and disadvantages of synthetic pesticides

Advantages of synthetic pesticides

- Often less expensive than an organic solution for a pest problem.
- Give longer periods of protection and less frequent and lower volumes of pesticide applied, saving time and money.
- When label directions are followed, foods grown with synthetic pesticides do not contain harmful residues.
- Readily available and have a longer shelf life than most organics.
- Relieve the grower of the necessity of relying on time-sensitive purchases and applications of pesticides.

Disadvantages of synthetic pesticides

- Do not breakdown quickly, can cause environmental concerns or have harvest restrictions.
- Broad-spectrum and may harm beneficial insects like pollinators, predators, and parasitoids.
- This can lead to secondary explosions of other pests, making further control measures necessary.

Effectiveness

Both natural and synthetic pesticides are effective at managing disease & pests. However, their modes of action can differ greatly. They often result in a drastic difference in the length of time it takes to see the intended results. Pest management professionals often get requests from their organic clients to "use the good stuff" (meaning synthetic pesticide option). This comes after some frustration with dealing with an infestation longer than expected. Synthetic pesticides often act quickly because they are chemically engineered to target and disrupt specific biological functions within the intended pest. While natural or organic pesticides will also work if given enough time and patience. The down side with natural options is that it may require more visits and multiple applications to achieve the same result. Many folks who are dealing with a pest infestation, seem to prefer the issue to be resolved quickly. They are unwilling to wait for the organic materials to do their job.

How to choose

- Choosing between organic and synthetic conventional pesticides is rarely straightforward.
- Both types of pesticides have benefits and limitations.

- You must weigh these pros and cons to determine which type of pesticide best suits your disease management goals.
- Understanding this information will also help you to use a product appropriately and with successful results.

Safety issues in pesticide uses

Harmful effects of pesticides

Pesticides can cause three types of harmful effects –

1. Acute
2. Delayed
3. Allergic

1. Acute effects

- Those effects that occur immediately after the exposure within minutes or hours.
- There can be physical effects on the body like
- Mouth throat and stomach can be burned, making it difficult to eat and drink.
    - Lungs can be burned, making it difficult to breath.
    - Skin can itch, blister, or crack.
    - Eyes can be burned, causing temporary or permanent blindness.

2. Delayed effects

- Illnesses or injuries that do not appear immediately and may take years to become apparent.
- They are caused by repeated exposure to a pesticide, pesticide group, or combination of pesticides over a long period of time.
- Delayed effects include cancer and other damage to internal organs.

3. Allergic effects

- Reactions that some people, but not all, develop after exposure to pesticides.
- For example, some people suffer from hay fever due to pollen in the air, while others do not.
- Allergic effects usually require several exposures before they become apparent.
- Typical reactions are asthma (difficulty in breathing), skin irritation (rashes, blisters, open sores), or eye and nose irritation (itchy, watery eyes and sneezing).

General symptoms and signs of pesticide poisoning

The typical symptoms and signs of pesticide poisoning are:

1. Initial

- Headache, dizziness.
- General weakness or tiredness.
- Nausea, vomiting.
- Tightness in chest.

2. Later

- Excessive sweating, salivation.
- Vomiting, diarrhoea.
- Stomach cramps.
- Muscle twitches, cramps, aches.
- Blurred vision.
- Confusion.
- Fits or unconsciousness.

13

Safety Issues in Pesticide Uses

I. First Aid

First aid is the initial treatment of a person suffering from a pesticide exposure, before seeking proper medical attention. The **first action** is to remove the person from the source of the exposure by removing pesticide from the skin, removing contaminated clothing, or getting the person to fresh air. While doing this, be careful to avoid contaminating yourself.

1. Pesticide on the skin

- Drench skin and clothing with plenty of water.
- Remove contaminated clothing.
- Wash hair and skin with soap and water.
- Dry the victim, and wrap in a blanket or any clean clothing. Do not allow the victim to become chilled or overheated.
- If the skin is burned, or injured, cover immediately with a loose, clean, dry, soft cloth or bandage.
- Do not apply ointments, greases or powders to burns or injured skin.
- Follow label instructions if available.

2. Pesticide in the eye

- Wash the eye(s) quickly but gently.
- Hold the eyelid open and wash with a gentle drip of water flowing across the eye rather than directly onto it.
- Rinse for 10 minutes or more.
- Do not use chemicals in the rinse water.
- Follow label instructions if available.

3. Pesticide inhaled

- Get the victim to fresh air immediately.
- Warn other people in the area of the danger.
- Loosen tight clothing that would restrict breathing.
- Follow label instructions if available.

4. Pesticide in mouth or swallowed

- Repeatedly rinse mouth with plenty of water.
- Do not induce vomiting if you can get the victim to a doctor within one hour.
- Never induce vomiting if the victim is unconscious or having convulsions.
- Never induce vomiting if the victim has swallowed a corrosive poison, as it will burn the throat and mouth as severely coming up as it did going down. It may also get into the lungs and cause burning there.
- Similarly, never induce vomiting if an emulsifiable or oil solution has been swallowed, as these can cause death if inhaled during vomiting.
- Apply artificial respiration if breathing has stopped or if the victim's skin is blue. If pesticide is on the victim's mouth or face, avoid direct contact during artificial respiration.
- Following the first aid, the victim must be taken to a doctor as quickly as possible, with the pesticide container or label so that the doctor can identify the active ingredient and follow label instructions if available.

II. Personal protective clothing

Protective clothing consists of clothing and devices that are worn to minimise exposure to pesticides and to keep pesticides away from the body. Protective clothing only protects if the pesticide remains on the outside and does not come into contact with the body. If pesticide gets inside the protective clothing, it holds the pesticide next to the body. Contaminated clothing should be removed immediately. All protective clothing should be cleaned at the end of every use. The minimum amount to wear for a specific pesticide formulation and activity is given on the label, either in the text or the pictograms.

Body protection

- When pesticides are handled, the minimum to wear is overalls.
- The collar should be fastened to protect the lower part of the neck. An alternative to overalls is a long sleeved shirt and long legged trousers. The shirt collar should be fastened to protect the lower part of the neck, the sleeves down and the cuffs buttoned.
- A wide brimmed, cotton or canvas hat can be worn during spraying to protect the head.
- All work clothes, including hats, should be washed after every days use.

Hand and foot protection

- Rubber gloves and rubber boots should be worn when handling pesticide concentrates. They should be unlined, as fabric liners can trap pesticide and are impossible to clean adequately.
- Trousers should be worn outside the boots, and not tucked in.

- Gloves should be washed with soap and water before removal, turned inside out and the inside washed. Boots should also be washed inside and out after use.
- Do not use gloves with holes or tears, as the pesticide will get inside and be held next to the skin.

Eye and face protection

- Non-fogging eyewear such as safety glasses and goggles should be worn when there is a chance of mists or dusts, for example during spraying or mixing dry formulations.
- Face shields should be worn when there is a risk of being splashed with insecticide, such as when mixing liquid formulations.
- An alternative is to use ordinary glasses or sunglasses. However, these give only minimal protection to the eyes.

Inhalation protection

- Dust/mist masks are usually shaped filters that cover the nose and mouth to filter out dusts, mists and particles.
- Masks must be disposed of after each days use.
- For spraying operations only, an alternative is a cloth tied over the nose and mouth. This should be washed after every spraying operation.

III How to safely use pesticides?

1. Take every safety precautions when using synthetic pesticides.
2. Don't use pesticides inside your house.
3. Users should be trained to use pesticides.
4. Read all of the safety instructions.
5. Check your local laws regarding pesticide use.
6. Never touch any pesticide chemicals with your bare skin.
7. Keep the right contact numbers ready.
8. Don't eat around pesticides.
9. Don't smoke around pesticides.
10. Keep pesticides away from children.
11. Don't assume that you are eliminating any risks just because you use natural pesticides.

14

Survey, Surveillance and Forecasting of Diseases

Definition

Sampling: Disease assessment activity within plots and fields.

Survey: To move over a specific place for some observation.

Surveillance: Repeated or sequential survey of some place/ locality for some observation to ascertain the changes /fluctuations in the objects of study.

Principle of survey

Principle of survey relates that no management practice should be followed against a pest unless its presence is confirmed at the population level that exceeds the economic threshold to make the management tactics economically desirable.

Objectives of survey

(1) To know the prevalence of disease in a crop in a particular area.

(2) To study the damages caused by a particular disease and assess the economic importance of the disease.

(3) To correlate the disease incidence with the weather factors, vegetation and soil factors.

(4) To give suitable forecasting to the farmers about the outbreak of file disease.

(5) To device suitable management strategies in advance by cultural and chemical means.

Kinds of survey

1) **Qualitative survey**: includes identification of different diseases.

2) **Quantitative survey**: involves the estimation of level of diseases or extent of losses due to disease .

Types of survey

1) **Random:** Samples are collected from any crop at any place suspected to be infested.

2) **Planned:** It is further of two types

a. **Extensive survey:** A vast area is taken in to consideration to obtain a preliminary assessment of disease.

b. **Intensive survey:** A particular area is surveyed to obtain accurate and detailed knowledge about the disease.

Methods of survey

(i) Fixed plot survey

- Select two villages and fix two fields per village.
- Select five sampling plots per field of one acre and it should be three metres away from the bunds.
- The size of the sample plot should be 1 sq, m.
- Select 20 plants or leaves per plot and observe for the disease intensity using the standard disease score chart having 0-9 grades.
- Work out the percent disease index(PDI)using the standard formula.
- Survey the field every week and prepare the report.

(ii) Roving survey

- Select four villages and in each village, fix two fields.
- Observe and score 1 00 plants or leaves in each field by walking across, starting from south west corner to north east corner.
- Work out the PDI using the standard formula.
- Survey the fields every week and prepare the report.

Design of Survey

- An impression of the health situation of an area or country can be obtained only be means of a survey.
- In a survey, fields to be sampled are selected so that together they represent the whole area.
- The design of the survey is not easy because it requires a compromise among various requirements, such as following
  - **Good statistical sampling**: The samples of fields is representative for the whole area.
  - **Transportation of personel**: Since the observers have to visit the sample fields.
  - **Time**: A survey having value only when a large area is covered within a short period.
  - **Money**: As surveys tend to be costly.

Requirement for successful survey

The essential requirement for success are

1. Record forms

- All forms should be readily understood and convenient for use in the field and for office processing.
- Only information known to the respondents, and which they are prepared to give, should be sought.
- Good questionnaires are brief, if there are many questions, the quality of information suffers.

2. Selection of staff , training and supervision

- Quality of staff must be appropriate to the work.
- All surveyors should be trained enough to know exactly what is expected of them and why.
- Adequate supervision is also needed to ensure that difficulties are resolved and a good standard of work maintained.

3. Establishing contact –public relations

- Effort must be made on the collaboration of farmers and local officials to secure their trust and interest.
- This can be done by advance publicity through digital media.

4. Data processing and reporting

- Before a survey is start, a plan should be made for processing the data and ensuring the essential clerical and computing facilities.
- Coding and computing should be carefully checked, because errors at this stage can invalidate much useful work.
- Consideration should be given to reporting of the results back to local officials and participating farmers by regional reports or discussion meetings.

5. Sample

- Sample must be sufficient to provide estimates to required accuracy.
- Survey should provide information from truly representative samples of the region under study, not just from farms convenient to visit or known to the extension services.

6. Method of observation and measurement

- Methods used by the field staff are consistent and reproducible and as objective as possible.
- Methods must be also acceptable to the farming community.

7. Disease Surveillance Reports

(i) **White report** : It contains the disease/pest surveillance detail in a particular block/division/district for a week.

(ii) **Yellow card** : It should be sent when the disease/pest occurrence attained half the level of economic threshold level (ETL).

(iii) **Red card** : It should be sent when the disease/pest occurrence exceeded the economic threshold level.

The weekly data on disease incidence along with the weather parameters collected from fixed plot and roving surveys are reported to the Joint Director of Agriculture in each district. These data collected from the farmers'fields and research centres in the district are pooled and interpreted jointly by the plant protection scientists of the University and Deputy Director of Agriculture (Plant Protection) every week and the action to be taken is decided. After analysing the weekly survey reports and the data on the weather factors, the message on the severity level of disease and management practices to be adopted are disseminated to the farmers through mass media. So surveillance and monitoring methods must be continuously adopted to trace the diseases, their movement and spread with a view to prevent the epidemics.

Pilot survey and Pre test

- A pilot survey, under similar conditions to those of the main survey, is essential, to check all aspects of the plan and obtain realistic estimates of the time and resources needed.
- It should be done soon enough for necessary modifications and for retraining.
- Pilot survey is impracticable for small survey (50 or so).

Aerial Survey

- Aerial survey can be of use when
  - Early infection foci have to be located.
  - Sudden disaster must be assessed immediately.
  - The terrain is inaccessible or the area too large.
- In these cases, ground survey is not satisfactory.
- Aerial photography in black and white is already classical; the same is true for black and white infrared sensitive film.
- Color film sensitivity to near infrared reflected radiation has given excellent results in some cases.
- Advanced techniques such as multispectral scanning (MSS), together with a good deal of computer science have been used.
- Aerial survey can be used for the purpose of disease detection, disease assessment, yield and loss assessment.

Disease Forecasting

Definition

Disease forecasting involves all the activities in ascertaining and notifying the grower community that conditions are sufficiently favourable for certain diseases, that application of control measures will result in economic gain or on the other hand , and just as important that the amount expected is unlikely to be enough to justify the expenditure of time, energy and money for

Types of forecast

Positive forecast: Employs need based chemical sprays, provides adequate protection to crop and reduces damage to environment.

Negative forecast: Avoids unnecessary chemical sprays, no risk to the crop health and no disruption of environment.

Importance of forecasting

- Forecasting informs the growers whether the conditions are not favourable and the disease is unlikely to be intense enough.
- This helps growers to save the expenditure in terms of energy, time and money by not applying unnecessary management measures.
- It informs the growers about when the conditions are going to be sufficiently favourable for economically important diseases of an agroclimatic zone.
- This help growers to apply disease management timely that results in economic gain.
- It helps growers to plan advance preventive measures against likely losses due to the occurrence of economically important severe diseases.
- Government and other organizations initiate necessary steps for the timely stocking of chemicals, equipments, etc. when they are timely warned by the possibility of an epidemic by the forecasting's.

Requirements for disease forecasting

The following requirements are necessary to make useful and successful disease forecasts

- The disease must cause economically significant damage in terms of yield loss or quality.
- Control measures must be available at an economically acceptable cost.
- Disease should not be regular feature.
- Grower must have adequate manpower and equipments to apply management measures when disease warning is given.
- Reliable means of communication with farmers.
- Farmers should be adaptive and have purchase power.

Information's needed for disease forecasting

The information's required for forecasting are:

1. Host factors

a. Prevalence of susceptible varieties in the given locality.
b. Response of host at different stages of the growth to the activity of pathogen.
c. Density and distribution of the host in a given locality.

2. Pathogen factors

a. Amount, of primary inoculum in the air, soil or planting material
b. Dispersal of inoculums
c. Spore germination
d. Infection
e. Incubation period
f. Sporulation on the infected host
g. Re-dispersal / Dissemination of spores
h. Perennating stages
i. Inoculum potential and density in the seed, soil and air

3. Environmental factors

a. Temperature
b. Humidity
c. Light intensity
d. Wind velocity

Methods of disease forecasting

Usually, the following methods are employed in disease forecasting.

1. Forecasting based on amount of initial inoculum

- Disease prediction can be made on the basis of amount of primary inoculums present in seed , soil or vector.
- This criterion is more vital for monocyclic diseases where amount of primary inoculums is related to disease severity and damage and secondary infection does not takes place.
- It is mostly used in case of loose smut of wheat and soil borne disease caused by Rhizocotnia, Sclerotium, Fusarium, Verticillium and Nematodes

2. Forecasting based on weather conditions

- The major criteria for diseases forecasting for polycyclic diseases is based on prevailing weather conditions *viz.*, temperature, relative humidity, rainfall, light, wind velocity etc.,
- Here in addition to amount of primary inoculums, the multiplication and dispersal of secondary inoculums are weather dependent.
- Forecasting of late and early blight of potato, wheat rust, anthracnose, apple scab, powdery mildew of cucurbits and downy mildew of grapes are made considering the prevailing weather conditions which determine the amount of disease and damage of the crop.

3. Forecasting based on correlative information

- Weather data of several years are collected and correlated with the intensity of the diseases.
- The data are compared and then the forecasting of the disease is done.
- Forecasting criteria developed from comparisons of disease observation with standard meteorological data have been provided for diseases like fire blight of apple and powdery mildew of barley.

4. Use of computer for disease forecasting

- Forecasting of disease is made by the use of computers in some developed countries
- The computers are fed with weather data collected on the farm by individual farmers.
- The computer then processes the data, determines whether an infection period is imminent, likely to occur or can not occur.
- A recommendation is made to the farmer as to whether or not to spray and what materials to apply. This system gives the results quickly.
- One such computer based programmes in the USA is known as 'Blitecast' for potato late blight.

Examples

a. Late blight of potato

Late blight of potato had been instrumental in development of diverse fundamental concepts in plant pathology and disease forecasting is no exception.The potato growers in Europe were intelligent enough to recognize blight weather (Moderate temperature and lots of moisture: rain, dew or humidity) much earlier than Van Everdingen postulated Dutch rules in 1926. Followings are four conditions correlated with weather that could predict about appearance of late blight in Netherlands:

- Night temperature below dew point at least 4 hours.
- Mainimum temperature of 10^{0}C or slightly above.
- Clouds on the next day.
- Rainfall during next 24 hours of at least 0.1 mm.

Notable contributions in late blight forecasting

- Van Everdingen postulated Dutch rules in 1926
- Krause, *et al.* (1970), BLITECAST
- Singh, *et al.* (1980), JHULSACAST for Indo Gangetic plains
- Fry and Apple (1983), Integrated host resistance and fungicide weathering in BLITECAST
- Dommermuth (1988), Phytoprog I. Late blight warning service
- Runno and Kopple (2002), NEGFRY
- Grunwald (2002), Modified and validated SIMCAST

Negative forecast

- When action and warning thresholds can be determined, it is also possible to determine that no action needs to be taken, at least within a certain period of time is called negative forecasting.
- An official negative forecasting system is operated in Germany for potato late blight under the name PHYTOFROG. BLITECAST also contains the option of negative forecasts.
- Negative forecasting system will become more popular in the future
- For example, cereal crops, particularly rice and wheat, are treated increasingly against various diseases. However, because of the relatively low margin of profit and the very large acreages involved, negative forecasts can prevent control costs from exceeding the limits of economy as well as forestall long term, unpredictable environmental and health hazards from chemical.

Supervised control

- It is the form of disease management system often, but not always, relying on the application of pesticides under the direction of a specialist.
- It is generally based on the assessment of disease intensity, crop loss and other ecological considerations.
- Since supervised control aims at the most efficient and least hazardous use ofchemicals , it is an essential component of many integrated control systems.
- BLITECASTS is a more advanced form of supervised control.
- Supervised control is more common in fruit growing areas and in large states where specialized supervisors are available.

15

Technologies and Services Required for Integrated Disease Management

A broad range of products and services are required by farmers in order to adopt Integrated Disease Management , calling for close interaction between them, the scientists and the experts developing IDM technologies. IDM must be based on farmers' concerns and circumstances. Farmers themselves are often the best judges of what is the most appropriate technology for their needs but the farmer's options may be limited due to government intervention, targeted, judicious and appropriate use of technologies protect and enhance the environment and contributes to sustainable production. The technologies and services required for IDM are

1. Field application.
2. Economic or action thresholds.
3. Sampling methods.
4. Conserving beneficials.
5. Novel products and techniques.
6. Resistance management.
7. Biotechnology.
8. Product research and development.
9. Improved application methods.
10. Season-long IDM crop programmes.
11. Pre-testing IDM methods and programmes.

1. Field application

Development and testing of farmer-oriented whole season crop programmes which may include:

- Crop calendar and critical stages for disease control.
- Disease complexes.
- Weather patterns.
- Identification of appropriate prevention, observation and intervention measures.
- Application techniques.

2. Economic or action thresholds

- It is important to monitor disease levels in a crop and only treat those which cause economic damage.
- It is important that thresholds are defined in a simple and understandable way so that farmers can adopt them in practice without undue difficulty.
- The economic or action thresholds may change depending on the stage of crop development, a range of biological and economic factors.
- Much work still needs to be done to develop accurate thresholds for the wide range of crops disease and environments that farmers have to deal with on a daily basis.

3. Sampling methods

- Farmers need simple methods for rapidly determining whether a disease in a crop is likely to cause economic damage.
- Guidance and support is needed to establish the effectiveness of different sampling procedures and related decision criteria.
- There are many ways in which local knowledge can be used to help develop practical methods acceptable to farmers.
- It is mandatory to develop local computerized databases to assist in making decisions on an area wide basis .

4. Conserving beneficials

- Conserving natural enemies of disease is recognized as an important part of IDM programmes.
- The impact of crop protection products on important beneficial microroganims needs to be monitored as a basis for developing appropriate IDM strategies.
- This should take account of the natural regulation of pathogen populations and their dynamics.
- The impact on important natural enemies also needs to be considered.
- Reductions in the amount of product used through IDM practice may reduce the exposure of natural enemies and lessen the risk of pest resurgence.

5. Novel products and techniques

- The continued search for novel modes of action of chemical and new biotechnology products will widen the range of IDM strategies and practices available to farmers and others managing diseases economically and sustainability.

6. Resistance management

- IDM offers a combination of tools, which reduce the risk that resistance will develop in pathogen populations.

- Monitoring the development of pathogen populations and applying treatments when the economic threshold is exceeded and implementing strategies such as alternating or mixing compatible crop protection products with different modes of action.
- A grower should utilise all tools available to avoid development of resistance.
- These tools include chemical and biological fungicides but also any agronomic practices that would reduce disease level or pathogen populations, such as crop rotation or reducing crop residues at the end of the season. The institutions can provide the information, but the grower must make the final decision.

7. Biotechnology

- Biotechnology has considerable potential to contribute to sustainable biological component of IDM.
- One focus of biotechnology research has been on improving natural enemies of diseases as disease control agents.
- This has focused principally on pathogens of diseases and their use as formulated biological pesticides.
- The second and most rapidly expanding area of biotechnology for disease control has been the development of crop varieties resistant to diseases, through genetic engineering, along with strategies for their sustainable use.

8. Product research and development

- Searching for and developing chemical, natural, biological and biotechnology products which widen the range of technologies available for IDM programmes.
- Investigating methodologies for incorporating new and existing products into IDM strategies.
- Developing decision-making tools such as diagnostics and forecasting system.

9. Improved application methods

- Timely and targeted application of plant protection products is an essential element of efficient disease control.It requires the use of appropriate and well maintained equipment and knowledge of the disease.
- Even simple changes (e. g. by directing the nozzle or lance to spray more where the disease is located, on the undersides of leaves or control of pressure at the nozzle) can improve spray coverage and give better management of a disease.
- Many farmers spray late or alter the dose because of difficulties in obtaining sufficient water to spray, especially in semi-arid and arid areas. There are reduced volume techniques available that allow farmers to treat more quickly when the disease level reaches the economic threshold. Ex.Drone

- Seed dressing, particularly with a systemic product that is transported throughout the plant, offers another solution to inefficient application , and also minimizes impacts on non-target organisms.
- There is a need to support changes in application efficiency rather than accept that farmers will only use the equipment currently on sale in the market place.

10. Season-long IDM crop programmes

- Research to determine the most suitable crop protection products, appropriate local dosage and timely recommendations during the crop season, needs close collaboration amongst scientists, as well as farmers, developing IPM in a particular farming area.
- Instead of recommending a number of separate products against individual disease, IDM may require a programme designed for a crop in a given area.
- The aim is to have season-long recommendations including products that complement other IDM tactics and provide a means of resistance management.

11. Pre-testing IDM methods and programmes

- It is important to understand farmers' perceptions of the disease problems and current practices of disease management.
- Socio-economic research is required to assess the acceptability and applicability of IDM recommendations.
- IDM recommendations must be flexible enough to adjust to changes in the environment, cropping patterns and market forces.
- It is important to understand the wider socio-economic effects of IDM programmes and the components they use.

16

Validation and Promotion of IDM Technologies

Validation of IDM technologies

Validation of IDM technologies is ultimate test for IDM knitted with available technologies under ground realities of the field. Since IDM is multidisciplinary, multi-organizational and multi-locational participatory approach, involvement of all the stakeholders, including farmers and field technicians is to be ensured. The following guidelines have been used as spirit behind the methodology of IDM validation.

1. Definitions and analysis of disease problems
2. Formulation of IDM modules
3. Selection of farmers
4. Collection of base line information
5. Orientation phase
6. Farmers' Field School (FFS)
7. Provision of vital IDM inputs
8. Impact analysis

1. Definitions and analysis of disease problems

- It is essential to survey the selected area to gather information on crops, varieties, crop production and protection practices followed by the farmers for managing the diseases.
- An analysis of the cropping systems, disease problems and their characteristics is essential.
- Historical data can also be useful in the process of defining the key disease problems.

2. Formulation of IDM modules

- Based on available information on the disease management tactics in that area, IDM modules are synthesized.
- Farmers practices are also kept in mind while synthesizing the IDM modules, which are expected to be eco friendly as well as farmer friendly.

3. Selection of farmers

- The selection of farmers to participate in an IDM programme, which is new to them, is not an easy task in initial stages and it needs sustained persuasion to convince the farmers that IDM will be good for them.
- Community participation is essential for the success of IDM.
- Once IDM succeeds with few farmers in the beginning itself, other farmers are then more likely to join the programme in the succeeding years.
- Identification and use of key farmers for spreading in IDM message is effective.

4. Collection of base line information

- Baseline data about the village and the participating farmers need to be collected.

5. Orientation phase

- This phase includes interaction with the farmers about the crops, varieties, disease problems, production and protection practices and the constraints in raising crop yields.
- Chart, photographs, pamphlets and audiovisual aids are used to attract the attention of the farmers towards improved crop varieties, modern production practices, key diseases, natural enemies of the diseases and the IDM practices to be validated.
- The farmers are explained about why, when and how of IDM in relation to the existing practices.
- The new IDM technologies , particularly the use of biocontrol inputs.

6. Farmers' Field School (FFS)

- Once farmers have adopted the programme, regular interactions with them through FFS at least once a week during the crop season is crucial.
- Day, time and venue for the FFS are prefixed.
- Usually, crop fields are used as "class rooms" to monitor the crop, diseases, natural enemies and take appropriate decisions for action.
- The farmers are encouraged to take up the leadership of FFS under the supervision of the scientists/ field technicians.

7. Provision of vital IDM inputs

- Availability of the critical inputs like seed , biopesticides, quality chemical pesticides, application equipments and protecting clothing for the safe use of pesticides is to be ensured.
- It has also been observed that small and marginal farmers are attracted to adopt new practices, if critical inputs are made available to them.

8. Impact analysis

- The standard impact assessment format are used to collect data, which are analyzed to find out impact of IDM on crop yields, biodiversity and profitability.
- Simple, farmer friendly and cost effective IDM modules are selected and recommended for dissemination in similar areas.

Promotion of Validated IDM Technologies

It is necessary to elaborate a dissemination strategy for horizontal spread of IDM technologies in wider areas, which have crop/disease problems similar to the location where IDM technology was validated. Essential components of the dissemination strategy are

1. Community participation
2. Training and education
3. Public-private sectors partnership
4. Availability of IDM inputs
5. Removal of obstacles in IDM implementation

1. Community participation:

- Success of IDM programme depends on the active participation of the farmers and village institutions.
- Participation and motivation of the women facilitates adoption. Area wide approach is essential to provide visible impacts of IDM.

2. Training and education

- As IDM is knowledge intensive, development of necessary human resources at all levels is required.
- Training of master trainers, extension personel, field technicians and the farmer to make them fully aware of the IDM concepts and philosophy; methodologies for prevention, monitoring and management of diseases;and decision making tools should be achieved.
- Appropriate training of the dealers/retailers of chemical pesticides/biopesticides is also required.
- For the participatory farmers, regular training through organizing Farmers Field Schools is considered mandataory.

3. Public-private sectors partnership

- Participation of ICAR institutes, State Agricultural Universities , Non Governmental Organizations and industries along with the farming families is effective for IDM implementation and deserves emphasis in the implementation strategy.

4. Availability of IDM inputs

- Timely supply of essential IDM inputs like seed, quality biocontrol agents etc is indispensable.
- Both public and private agencies are expected to ensure that the essential IDM inputs are made available to the farmers on time.

5. Removal of obstacles in IDM implementation

- For effective IDM programme implementation it is essential to be able to address the key problems.
- Farmers think that the chemical pesticides are easy to apply and act quickly and their success can be seen immediately. Holistic IDM is relatively complex as it requires knowledge of the complex interrelationships within the agro ecosystem and demands a farsighted planning.

17

Implementation, Adoption and Scaling up of IDM Strategies

The eventual objective of promoting IDM is to empower its users to engage sustainable agricultural production with long term positive impacts on human being, poverty and environmental health.The impact of successful implementation of IDM approaches cannot be achieved if IDM is not strategically placed within national policies for agricultural production and protection. There are number of the national policies and related regulations that have direct impact on IDM adoption and scaling up in India.

This would cover:

1. Pest/disease management policies
2. Judicious use of pesticides
3. Plant quarantine
4. Seed certification
5. Education and training policy
6. Technology transfer and capacity building
7. Public and private sector partnership

1. Disease/Pest management policies

- IDM-promoting policies like sustaining disease surveillance, establishment of regional and national forecasting and early warning systems, decision support systems need to be promoted .
- These policies implemented by Ministries of Agriculture in and endeavor to reduce yield losses

2. Judicious use of pesticides

- Pesticides are going to play a major role till we perfect other disease control options.
- Pesticide use should be selective and need based. .
- There is a great need to make farmers aware about pesticide application technology.
- Use of ICT will facilitates safe and judicious use of pesticides and will also reduce the pesticide load in the environment and subsequent residue problems

3. Plant quarantine

- Quarantine forms the basis for transboundaary disease prevention through control of sources of disease introduction and incursions.
- Disease surveys and pest risks analysis (PRA) studies are critical for preparing and updating quarantine disease lists.
- Early detection and reporting of the introduction or emergence of a new disease through regular surveys is indispensable for checking disease spread before it reaches epidemic levels.
- Quarantine needs to be supported with financial, human and infrastructural resources.

5. Seed certification

- Use of clean seed /planting material would be a prime component of any IDM programme.
- National policies allied to the quality control, availability and cost of inputs for farmers is vital for IDM adoption.
- This encompasses systems for inspection and certification of seeds and vegetative material and nursery control.
- Such policies need to be properly assessed and designed in terms of their economic feasibility practicality and accessibility to farmers could be a support to IDM programmes.
- This is particularly true in India where subsistence farmers may not be able to afford the cost of certified seeds and seedlings or have inadequate transportation access to source of seeds.

5. Education and training

Education and training skills are required by farmers to adopt and implement IDM. These include:

- Recognition of diseases, antagonists and their uses.
- How to keep initial disease pressure low using every farm management opportunity?
- How to select the most suitable cultivars to grow?
- How to assess the importance of level of diseases and crop damage, as a low disease pressure may not cause economic damage?
- How to select which crop protection products to use; with emphasis on efficacy to the target disease, user and environmental safety, specificity on the target disease, and resistance management strategy?
- How to monitor for resistance?
- How to decide when to apply a crop protection product?

- Where crop protection products are needed; and if treatments can be localized?
- What equipment is needed to apply the product?
- How to calibrate equipment?
- What safety precautions are needed for applicators others and the environment?

6. Technology transfer and capacity building

- Long-term and sustainable adoption of IDM by farmers will only occur if the information and knowledge of technology and strategy are made available to them.
- A sense of "ownership" for that strategy by the farmers as well as local governmental and non-governmental organizations is also key.
- An essential element towards achieving this is providing access to information and training that can enhance the capacity of these groups to implement the strategies effectively and further develop and adapt them to local conditions.
- The public and private sector institutes are actively engaged in training and capacity building programmes across the country which provide the knowledge required to apply IDM practically and use the range of products available effectively.

7. Public and private sector partnership

- The private sector is profit-driven and highly competitive, concentrating on return on investment and based on shareholder capital.
- The public sector is non-profit and non competitive, concentrating on socio-economic investment and based on social and human capital.
- There is a common ground, however, public-sector institutions promote an environment in which the economy thrives by fostering human development, social cohesion and good governance.
- The private sector increasingly acknowledges that without social infrastructure, education, health, access to clean water and arable land, no stable political and enabling environment can be guaranteed, and this, in turn, affects the private sector "bottom line".
- There is recognition of the need to address the "triple bottom line" – social, environmental, and economic factors – if the goals of sustainable development and sustainable business are to be realized.
- The public sector is coming to realize that the private sector is a driving force behind growth and that it should not be overlooked when poverty alleviation initiatives are being formulated.
- A more lasting impact could be achieved if poverty was addressed by building on each partner′s competencies and comparative advantages and by creating long-term relationships through the expansion of successful partnerships in both scope and geographic coverage.

How is IDM Implemented?

IDM uses all suitable techniques or strategies to keep diseases below levels that cause unacceptable crop loss. These different strategies are usually placed under the main headings of mechanical, cultural, sanitation, biological, and chemical methods of disease management.

There are many individual methods under these headings which can be used in an IDM programme. Those which are actually used will depend on the crop and disease situation, and also to some extent on the infrastructure under which the crop is produced, as well as the availability of resources.

Any crop is a dynamic system – it is constantly changing. It is changing within a season due to the natural growth stages of the crop (seedling, vegetative, reproductive stages), as a result of the farmers management practices (thinning, weeding, fertilizer application, irrigation etc) and as a result of changes in disease types and numbers. It also changes between seasons as one year may be generally hotter or cooler than another or one year may have more rainfall than another. The implementation of disease management needs to take this dynamic situation into account.

Essentials for implementation

1) Availability of location-specific IDM modules which are ecologically sound, economically viable and socially acceptable.
2) High level of target group participation.
3) Area-wide dissemination strategy.
4) Removal of obstacles in dissemination of IDM.
5) Measuring, evaluating and publicizing the impacts of IDM.

Steps in the Implementation of IDM

1. Correct disease identification.
2. Understanding of disease and crop dynamics.
3. Planning preventive strategies.
4. Monitoring.
5. Decision making.
6. Selection of optimal disease control tactics.
7. Implementation.
8. Evaluation.

1. **Correct disease identification** - what diseases/pests and stages are causing the damage. This is foundation of all decision making.
2. **Understanding of disease and crop dynamics** - We must have enough information about the nature of the pathogens encountered to assess the potential risk that the disease poses and determine the best possible management strategy.

- How much disease is tolerable?
- What are the expected losses of the disease if controls are not used?
- What is the most vulnerable stage for management?
- Two concepts of importance: window of vulnerability and treatment window

3. **Planning preventive strategies**: It is the preferred management strategy in IDM. A care full examination of field history and all aspects of the crop production system should be made to determine if the crop can be grown or treated to prevent disease form exceeding economic levels.
    - Can any agronomical practice like summer ploughing, time of sowing, crop rotation, fertilizer management, water management etc, be manipulated to reduce disease attack?
    - What are the existing natural control agents that can be augmented or conserved?
    - Are the chances of economic disease losses great enough to justify a preventive pesticide strategy?
    - What are the benefits and risks of pesticides?
4. **Monitoring**- It involves periodic assessment of diseases, natural control factors, crop characteristics, and environmental factors to be needed for management and the effectiveness of any management action. Different methods and sampling frequencies are used, depending on the nature of diseases and monitoring objective.
5. **Decision making**- An evaluation of the monitoring information to assess the relevant economic benefits versus the risks of disease management actions.
    - What will I lose if I do nothing? What will I gain?
    - Is there enough natural control agents present to reduce the disease incidence/ severity below economic levels?
    - Is the incidence/severity potential of the disease more costly than the management?
    - Estimate "economic thresholds" or "action thresholds" which serve as references for loss potential at particular crop growth stages or sets of crop conditions.
6. **Selection of optimal disease management tactics:** The disease management tactics should be selected to manage the disease while minimizing economic, health and environmental risks.
    - How well will the management option fit into the total management system?
    - How well will the tactics management the disease?
    - What effects will this action have on the end user, society as a whole , and the environment.?
    - Will this action impact, either positively or negatively on other species or

natural enemies present in crop?

- Are there opportunities to integrate nonchemical tactics?
- What is the best fungicide for the target disease? What is the optimal rate? Is it legal?
- What are the safety requirements and use restrictions?

7. **Implementation** – The selected management options should be deployed on a timely manner with precision and completeness.
   - What can be done to improve effectiveness of the management tactics?
   - If pescticide are used, what is the appropriated chemical and rate for the target pest?
   - Is the pesticide application equipment is in good condition and calibrated properly?
   - Can the pesticide applied in the manner that will be least disruptive on natural enemies while still provide effective management ?
   - It might be desirable to leave small non- treated areas to evaluate management effectiveness in certain situations.
9. **Evaluation** – Always take time to follow-up and evaluate disease management actions to determine if you got your money's worth. Review what went wrong but more importantly what went right.
   - Was the chance of management action appropriate?
   - What changes to the management tactics can be made to improve management if the same disease problem occurs in the future?
   - Was the management action implemented on time and according to recommendations?
   - What future changes in the production system can be made to achieve more permanent suppression of the disease problem?

Major obstacles in implementation of IDM

Major obstacles

Although, IDM has been acknowledged as the most attractive option for protection of crops from the ravages of diseases, but implementation at the farmers levels has been inadequate. Pesticide continue to dominate and their injurious use represents the greatest threat to IDM. For an effective implementation strategy, it is essential to identify the obstacles to its dissemination, some of which are

1. Inadequate interaction between research and extension agencies.
2. Low awareness and innovativeness of extension personnel and target groups.
3. Problem of timely and adequate supply of quality inputs, including biocontrol agents and biopesticides.
4. Complexity of IDM vs simplicity of chemical pesticides.

5. Dominant influence of pesticide industry.
6. Non-availability of location specific IDM module for many crops.

Adoption of IDM

Generally IDM approaches are location specific and knowledge intensive. Accordingly farmers or extensionists, would required to understand the agro-ecological processes affecting the disease and, accordingly, make informed decisions on how best to manage crops to avoid/prevent disease occurrence, as well as how to manage these diseases once they become a problem. .

The following points may be considered for increased adoption of IDM:

1. National policy.
2. Economic and regulatory measures.
3. Development of markets.
4. Farmer-centered research, extension and training.

1. National policy: Establishment of a national IDM policy framework is the first step in area wide adoption of IDM.The following are the key components of the IDM policy are

- Maintaining ecological balance.
- Executing appropriate action on pesticides.
- Operating an effective system for implementing the national IDM programme.
- Developing human resources as the core of IDM.
- Conducting research on IDM.

2. Economic and regulatory measures

- The financial impact of IDM policies like lower subsidies, licensing, taxes and registration fees fall most heavily on producers and marketers of pesticides and initially falls most heavily on producers of cash crops.
- Tax exemptions and subsidies on biopesticies can have a significant impact on the the adoption of IDM.

3. Development of markets

- Of late, market for pesticide free or organic food has been growing fast.
- Consumers are becoming aware, better informed and are even indicating preferences for low pesticide residue products.
- Consumers' awareness need to backed up by dependable standards and labeling procedures.
- India could be good prospects for development of potentially lucrative export market of organic product if can establish and maintain quality.

- Attentions should be paid to preferential treatments, long term contracts and quality preferences.
- In the long-run, export markets of India is expected to be more pesticide-sensitive.

4. Farmer centered research, extension and training

- Intensive research is needed to standardize the IDM packages for different crops.
- Farmers, extension workers and local crop protection technicians should have practical understanding of the ecology and disease cycle of major diseases and their antagonists and this knowledge be translated into appropriate decision making tools and practical control tactics.
- A widespread extension and training programme should be launched for farmers, extension workers and local crop production technicians.
- Training should be backed by a continuous flow of information from scientists, farmers and others. This information could be transmitted on daily or weekly basis.
- Support of IDM implementation is inconsistent with a top –down technology transfer approach.
- Farmers to farmers exchanges with success stories using biological controls and IDM would help in disseminating to other farmers.
- Some selected farmers could even be provided financial support to educate and train other farmers to strengthen implementation of IDM.
- Demonstration of socio-economic benefits of IDM on a large scale for its horizontal spread.

Constraints in adoption of IDM

- Farmers are addicted to subsidy. They always look for some financial support for adopting IDM technologies.
- Biopesticides, disease resistant varieties and other IDM components are not readily available.
- There is few government machinery to monitor the quality of biopesticcides so, the desired results are not observed in many cases.
- Large farmers discourage small farmers in adopting IDM technologies by emphasizing more on their risky and unstable nature.
- Scientific community is constrained in recommending use of IDM technology because farmers may ask for compensation in case of failures.
- Pesticide dealers pose a threat to IDM by offering seeds, fertilizers and pesticides on credit to the farmers.

Scaling-up of IDM Practices

The undernoted points may be considered for scaling-up of IDM practices

- Integrated disease management programmes required to be identified and established at an early stage of implementation linkages with individual or organizations that can provide mechanisms for future scaling up.
- Key institutions and persons should be involved in the design, planning, implementation and evaluation of the progrmme.
- Analysis of potential organizations like public, private, NGO etc that is vital for the scaling up .Their mandates, roles, responsibilities and capacities need to be assessed and strengthened on regular basis.
- Eliminating policies that promote environmentally unsustainable disease and pest management techniques.
- Implementation of positive measures to promote IDM with emphasis on decentralized, farmer-centered initiatives through support of research, extension and training.
- Awareness of decision makers at the national, state and districts levels for promotion of IDM.
- Decision makers should be able to visit and see an FFS first hand and talk directly with farmers.

18

Technological, Socio-economic, Institutional and Policy Issues of IDM

India has successfully reduced pesticide consumption without adversely affecting the agricultural productivity. This was facilitated by appropriate policies that discouraged pesticide use and favored IDM application. Despite it, adoption of IDM is low owing to a number of socio –economic, institutional and policy issues. The issues important in making IDM work under field conditions

1. Available technologies
2. Technical efficacy
3. Economic feasibility
4. Technology characteristics
5. Technology dissemination
6. Community participation
7. Supply of biopesticides
8. Enforcement of pesticide regulations
9. Economic incentives
10. Development of market for pesticide-free products

1. Available technologies

- The Directorate of Plant Protection&Quarantine, Ministry of Agriculture, Government of India, has evolved location specific IPM packages for both the kharif and rabi crops in consultation with IPM experts from the Indian Council of Agricultural Research, State Agricultural Universities, and the State Departments of Agriculture that may be referred.
- Some important commercially products include *Trichoderma*, *Pseudomonas*, and *Bacillus* etc. are available as biopesticides for end users at reasonable cost.
- Phytoproducts like azadirachtin, pyrethrum, nicotine etc are also available as biopesticides.

2. Technical efficiency

- IDM must be sound on technical and economic parameters .
- Change in the pesticide use and yield change over the conventional chemical

control are the two criteria on which basis technical feasibility of IDM should be judged .

- The basic goal of IDM is to reduce pesticde and this evidence is well established under field conditions.
- The effect of IDM on yield could be either way. However, evidences suggest that substantial yield saving advantage of IDM over chemical control in crops.

3. Economic feasibility

- IDM is a cost effective technology.
- The extent of net benefits though would depend on the type of input used in IDM package, its application rate and price.
- IDM has the potential to substitute chemical pesticides without having any adverse effects on agricultural productivity.
- Inputs prices are an important determinant of the economic feasibility of IDM and any increase in prices of vital inputs may disturb its economics.

4. Technology characteristics

- Characteristics of technologies have vital role in farmers adoption decisions.
- IDM is a complex technology depends heavily on complimentary interactions of diverse methods of disease management like cultural, mechanical, biological, chemical etc.
- Each of the component has its own specific characteristics and requirements for application.
- Generally, farmers adopt those components that show immediate effect, and are easily available.
- Biopesticdes comprise a major component of IDM. Most of the biopesticides are slow in action, host specific and have short shelf life. Besides application of some of the components is labour intensive compared to conventional chemical control.
- Such technological uniqueness create an apprehension among the farmring about their efficacy to control diseases.
- The complexicity of IDM necessitates active involvement of researchers, extension workers and farmers to alleviate apprehensions through participatory /adaptive research trials.
- Researchers need to do basic research for development of broad spectrum biopesticides and improvement in their efficacy and shelf life.
- Emphasis should also be given on development of bio-pesticides having, stable formulation, long shelf life, better compatibility with chemical pesticides.
- Biotechnology has got tremendous potentialities for developing biopesticides.

5. Technology dissemination

- IDM is knowledge intensive and akin to a new technology.
- It effective implementation needed extension workers to have a sound understanding of target host, natural enemies, toxicity, method of application, etc before the technology is delivered to the farmers. Lack of understanding of any of these would adversely affect its adoption.
- Extension worker should act more as a collaborator, consultant and facilitator in dissemination of the knowledge, with the farmer playing a more active role.
- Government should have to made considerable efforts to impart training to the extension worker in order to achieve the desired objectives.
- 'Farmers Field Schools' needs to be established more and more to transfer the skills to the farmers.
- Extension system required to overhauled in knowledge about IDM inputs, methodology of IDM and timely delivery of services to the farmers to accelerate the adoption of IDM.

6. Communityparticipation

- Community participation is key to successful adoption of IDM .
- It needs to be sustained by devising an appropriate policy.
- Local bodies like, panchayats, NGOs, self help groups, etc should be encouraged to shoulder the responsibility.
- Incentives and award should be given to those farmers who are following IDM approach.

7. Supply of biopesticides

- Supply of biopesticides is vital to sustainability of IDM.
- Indian biopesticide market is expected to deliver 778 million dollar by 2025 at a CAGR of 25.4%.
- Market share of biopesticides in India is about 4.5% of total pesticides sale.
- Fruit and vegetable segment are started shifting towards the biopesticides due to increasing food safety concerns from consumer end.
- Worldwide biopesticides market is projected to grow at a CAGR of 14.7% from an estimated value of 4.3 billion USD in 2020 to reach 8.5 billion USD by 2025.
- Global demand for biopesticides is increasing daily due to consumer awareness regarding food safety.
- Most of the biopesticides are not broad spectrum and are slow in action.
- Many of these like Trichoderma and Pseudomonas have short shelf life and production of bioesticides is fraught with risk.
- Expansion of biopesticides industry are uncertain due to unstable demand, lack of appropriate infrastructure for transportation, storage and marketing.

- Biopesticide manufacturing units are under strict registration and quality control requirements.
- The process of registration is costly and burdensome that discourages potential entrepreneurs .
- Educated youths and rural unemployed should be encouraged to establish small scale biopesticide production units at village and block level.
- To stimulate production of biopesticides, measures like provision of institutional credits, subsidies, training to the potential entrepreneurs, insurance against low off take of inputs due to low disease pressures and exemption from taxes and duties would be taken.
- Registration requirement should be relaxed, though without compromise with quality standard.

8. Enforcement of pesticide regulations

- It will help to improve adoption of IDM .
- Presence of spurious pesticides in the market results in losses of yield and farmers' income.
- 30% of plant protection chemicals sold in India are spurious
- There are more than 6,000 agro-chemical companies in India.
- Most of them are not running as per the guidelines of CIB&RC which allows prosecution – but it isn't happening.
- Use of spurious pesticides is growing at about 20% every year.
- Uttar Pradesh, Madhya Pradesh, Maharashtra, Andhra Pradesh, Karnataka, Haryana and West Bengal are among the worst-affected States.
- As per research done by Indian Institute of Public Administration with the help of Ministry of Consumer Affairs, 58% of agri inputs are fake in rural India.
- Government need to enforce strong regulations on production, use, distribution and quality of pesticides and weed out spurious elements, ultimately benefit the farmers.

9. Economic incentives

- Economic incentives should support farmers switching over to IDM practices.
- Price of technology is vital determinants in farmers's decision for its adoption.
- Government of India should think of classifying biopesticides into 'green box' for provision of subsidies.
- Withdrawal of subsidies on chemical pesticides and diversion of the same towards production and use of biopesticides .
- Linking of institutional credit and insurance with IDM adoption would induce farmers switching over to IDM.

10. Development of market for pesticide-free products.

- It is now obligatory to create awareness among consumers about benefits of organic produce for health.
- Presently, there are no first-rate markets and standards for organic food in India.
- Simple and cost effective certification and labeling systems required to be developed.
- It should enable farmers to produce pesticide free products and to gain confidence of the consumers and ultimately will boost adoption of IDM.

Strategies for adoption of Effective Disease Management

Following strategies could help to improve adoption of IDM:

- Development of biointensive and cost effective IDM practices by holistic integration of all the informations.
- Validation and promotion of IDM practices among stake holders.
- Improved availability of vital inputs like resistant varieties, planting materials, biopesticides etc.
- Development of the monitoring tool's and forewarning system.
- Training of farmers and extension personnel about IDM methodology.
- Intensive research on development of multiple disease and pest resistant varieties.
- Aggressive demonstration campaigns by R&D institutions in collaboration with state functionaries and non-governmental organizations (NGOs).
- Advocate use of green chemicals and ICT based application technologies.
- Urgent need for intensifying research on design and discovery of new green molecules would also support 'Make in India' program.
- Sale and use of spurious pesticides is indeed a real problem which needs to be addressed on priority.
- Come out with a generic policy on the chemicals that has lasting impact and promotes the growth of agriculture in the country.
- To foster innovation and modernization, there is an urgent need to adopt and implement advanced technologies for better, efficient and eco-friendly environment.

19

IDM in Important Crops

19.1 IDM in Rice

Sl.No	Major Diseases	Causal Organism
1	Blast	*Pyricularia oryzae*
2	Brown spot	*Helminthosporium oryzae*
3	Sheath blight	*Rhizoctonia solani*
4	Sheath rot	*Sarocladium oryzae*
5	False smut	*Ustilaginoidea virens*
6	Udbatta disease	*Ephelis oryzae*
7	Stem rot	*Sclerotium oryzae*
8	Bacterial leaf blight	*Xanthomonas oryzae pv. oryzae*
9	Bacterial leaf streak	*Xanthomonas oryzae pv. oryzicola*
10	Tungro (RTD)	*Rice tungro bacilliform virus* and *Rice tungro spherical virus*
11	Grassy stunt	*Rice grassy stunt tenuivirus*
12	Rice dwarf	*Rice dwarf virus*
13	Rice yellow dwarf	*Rice yellow dwarf virus*

1. Blast - *Pyricularia oryzae*

Diagnostic Symptoms

- Pathogen attacks the crop at all stages of crop growth.
- Symptoms appear on leaves, nodes, rachis, and glumes. On the leaves, the lesions appear as small bluish green flecks, which enlarge under moist weather to form the characteristic spindle shaped spots with grey centre and dark brown margin **(Leaf blast).**
- The spots coalesce as the disease progresses and large areas of the leaves dry up and wither. Severely infected nursery and field appear as burnt.
- Black lesions appear on nodes girdling them. The affected nodes may break up and all the plant parts above the infected nodes may die **(Nodal blast).**

- During flower emergence, the fungus attacks the peduncle and the lesion turns to brownish-black which is referred to as rotten neck / neck rot / panicle blast (**Neck blast**).
- In early neck infection, grain filling does not occur while in late infection, partial grain filling occurs.

2. Brown Spot - *Helminthosporium oryzae*

Diagnostic Symptoms

- Infected seedlings have small, circular, yellow brown or brown lesions that may girdle the coleoptile and distort primary and secondary leaves.
- Starting at tillering stage, lesions can be observed on the leaves.
- They are initially small, circular, and dark brown to purple-brown.
- Fully developed lesions are circular to oval with a light brown to gray center, surrounded by a reddish brown margin caused by the toxin produced by the fungi.
- Lesions on leaf sheaths are similar to those on the leaves.
- Infected glumes and panicle branches have dark brown to black oval spots or discoloration on the the entire surface.
- Spikelets can also be infected. Infection of florets leads to incomplete or disrupted grain filling and a reduction in grain quality.
- The disease-causing fungi can also penetrate grains, causing *'pecky rice'*, a term used to describe spotting and discoloration of grains.

3. Sheath Blight -*Rhizoctonia solani*

Diagnostic Symptoms

- Initial symptoms are noticed on leaf sheaths near water level.
- On the leaf sheath oval or elliptical or irregular greenish grey spots are formed.
- As the spots enlarge, the centre becomes greyish white with an irregular blackish brown or purple brown border.
- Lesions on the upper parts of plants extend rapidly coalesing with each other to cover entire tillers from the water line to the flag leaf.
- The presence of several large lesions on a leaf sheath usually causes death of the whole leaf, and in severe cases all the leaves of a plant may be blighted.
- The infection extends to the inner sheaths resulting in death of the entire plant.
- Plants heavily infected in the early heading and grain filling growth stages produce poorly filled grain, especially in the lower part of the panicle.
- The fungus affects the crop from tillering to heading stage.

4. Sheath Rot -*Sarocladium oryzae*

Diagnostic Symptoms

- Initial symptoms appear only on the upper most leaf sheath enclosing young panicles.
- The flag leaf sheath show oblong or irregular greyish brown spots.
- They enlarge and develop grey centre and brown margins covering major portions of the leaf sheath.
- The young panicles remain within the sheath or emerge partially.
- The panicles rot and abundant whitish powdery fungal growth is seen inside the leaf sheath.

5. False Smut - *Ustilaginoidea virens*

Diagnostic Symptoms

- Individual rice grain transformed into a mass of velvety spores or yellow fruiting bodies.
- Growth of velvety spores enclose floral parts.
- Immature spores slightly flattened, smooth, yellow, and covered by a membrane.
- Growth of spores result to broken membrane.
- Mature spores orange and turn yellowish green or greenish black.
- Only few grains in a panicle are usually infected and the rest are normal.

6. Udbatta - *Ephelis oryzae*

Diagnostic Symptoms

- Symptoms appear at the time of panicle emergence.
- The entire ear head is converted into a straight compact cylindrical black spike like structure.
- The spikelets are cemented to the central rachis and the size is remarkably reduced.
- The entire spike is covered by greyish stroma with convex pycnidia immersed inside.

7. Stem Rot - *Sclerotium oryzae*

Diagnostic Symptoms

- Small black lesions are formed on the outer and inner leaf sheath at the water line.
- Later on, these lesions gradually make their appearance on the inner leaf sheaths and the culm.
- Affected tissues rot and abundant small black sclerotia are seen in the rotting tissues.

- Culm collapses and plants lodge.
- Sclerotia are carried in stubbles after harvest.

8. Foot Rot or Bakanae -*Fusarium moniliforme*

Diagnostic Symptoms

- In the nursery, infected seedlings are lean and lanky, much taller and die after some time.
- In the main field, the affected plants have tall lanky tillers with longer internodes and aerial adventitious roots from the nodes above ground level.
- The root system is fibrous and bushy.
- The plants are killed before earhead formation or they produce only sterile spikelets.

9. Bacterial Leaf Blight -*Xanthomonas oryzae pv. oryzae*

Diagnostic Symptoms

- Wilting and yellowing of leaves, or wilting of seedlings (also called kresek).
- On seedlings, infected leaves turn grayish green and roll up.
- As the disease progresses, the leaves turn yellow to straw-colored and wilt, leading whole seedlings to dry up and die.
- Kresek on seedlings may sometimes be confused with early rice stem borer damage.
- To distinguish kresek symptoms from stem borer damage, squeeze the lower end of infected seedlings between the fingers.
- Kresek symptoms should show yellowish bacterial ooze coming out of the cut ends.
- Unlike plants infested with stem borer, rice plants with kresek are not easily pulled.
- On older plants, lesions usually develop as water-soaked to yellow-orange stripes on leaf blades or leaf tips or on mechanically injured parts of leaves. Lesions have a wavy margin and progress toward the leaf base.
- On young lesions, bacterial ooze resembling a milky dew drop can be observed early in the morning. The bacterial ooze later on dries up and becomes small yellowish beads underneath the leaf pulled out from soil.
- Old lesions turn yellow to grayish white with black dots due to the growth of various saprophytic fungi. On severely infected leaves, lesions may extend to the leaf sheath.

Quick diagnose bacterial blight on leaf:

- Cut a young lesion across and place in a transparent glass container with clear water.

- After a few minutes, hold the container against light and observe for thick or turbid liquid coming from the cut end of the leaf

10. Bacterial Leaf Streak -*Xanthomonas oryzae pv. oryzicola*

Diagnostic Symptoms

- Fine translucent streaks are formed on the veins and the lesions enlarge lengthwise and infect larger veins and turn brown.
- On the surface of the lesions, bacterial ooze out and form small yellow band-like exudates under humid conditions.
- In severe cases the leaves dry up.

11. Rice Tungro Disease (RTD) - *Rice tungro bacilliform virus* (RTBV) and *Rice tungro spherical virus* (RTSV)

Diagnostic Symptoms

- Plants are markedly stunted.
- Leaves show yellow to orange discoloration and interveinal chlorosis.
- Young leaves are sometimes mottled while rusty spots appear on older leaves.
- Tillering is reduced with poor root system.
- Panicles not formed in very early infection, if formed, remain small with few, deformed and chaffy grains.

12. Rice Grassy Stunt - *Rice grassy stunt tenuivirus*

Diagnostic Symptoms

- Plants severely stunted.
- Excessive tillering.
- Very upright plant growth.
- Grassy and rosette appearance of plants.
- Yellowish green leaves that are shorter and narrower than normal.
- Leaves that remain yellow even after application of sufficient nitrogen fertilizers.
- Numerous small rusty spots or patches on leaves, which merge into blotches.
- Leaves blotches have a mottled appearance.
- Plants that fail to produce panicles.

Crop stage wise IDM activities in Rice		
Crop stage	**Diseases**	**Step wise IDM practices**
Nursery	Soil borne pathogens	• Deep ploughing of fields during summer to control nematodes population, to expose popagules of soil borne pathogens. • Timely sowing should be done. • Balanced use of fertilizers and micro-nutrients as per local recommendations. • Seed treatment with carbendazim+ mancozeb 50% WP @ 2 g/kg seed or Trichoderma/Pseudomonas @ 5-10 g/ha of seed for seed or soil borne diseases. • Field sanitation. • Destroy the alternate host plants. • Crop rotation with non-cereals.
	Blast	• Use resistant/tolarent varieties. • Spray isoprothiolan 40% EC @ 750 ml/ha or tricyclo-zole 75% WP @ 300-400 g/ha
	BLB	• Use the tolerant varieties. • Chemical Control: Spray of streptomycin sulphate 9% + tetracycline hydrochloride 1% SP @ 100-150 ppm.
Vegetative stage	Blast	• Use resistant/tolarent varieties. • Spray isoprothiolan 40% EC @ 750 ml/ha or tricy-clozole 75% WP @ 300-400 g/ha or tricyclazole 70% WG @ 300 g/ha
	BLB	• Use the tolerant varieties. • Chemical Control: Spray of streptomycin sulphate 9% + tetracycline hydrochloride 1% SP @ 100-150 ppm. • Reduce nitrogen application and apply if needed only small dose of N in more split doses.
	Sheath blight	• Spray validamycin 3% L @ 2000 g/ha or hexaconazole 5% EC @ 1000 ml/ha or propiconazole 25% EC @750 ml/ha or propiconazole 10.7% + tricyclazole 34.2% SE @ 500 ml/ha..
	White tip nem-atode	• Sun drying of seeds for 6 hours for 4 days. • Pre-sowing of nursery bed treatment with carbofuran 3% CG @ 50 kg/ha if nematode population crosses the ETL.

	Root knot nematode	• Rotation with the crops like sweet potato, sunflower, cowpea, sesamum, and onion. • Soil application of carbofuran 3% CG @ 50 kg/h..
Panicle initiation to booting	Blast	• Same as in vegetative stage.
	BLB	• Same as in vegetative stage.
	Sheath blight	• Same as in vegetative stage.
Flowering stage	Blast	• Same as in vegetative stage.
	Sheath blight	• Same as in vegetative stage.

19.2 IDM inWheat

Sl.No	Major Diseases	Causal Organism
1	Loose smut	*Ustilago nuda tritici* (*Ustilago tritici)*
2	Black or stem rust	*Puccinia graminis tritici*
3	Brown or leaf rust	*Puccinia triticina (P. recondita)*
4	Yellow or stripe rust	*Puccinia striiformis*
5	Flag smut	*Urocystis tritici*
6	Hill bunt or stinking smut	*Tilletia caries / T.foetida*
7	Karnal bunt	*Neovossia indica*
8	Powdery mildew	*Erysiphe graminis var. tritici*
9	Leaf blight	*Alternaria triticina / Bipolaris sorokiniana*

1. Loose Smut -*Ustilago nuda tritici (Ustilago tritici)*

Diagnostic Symptoms

- Infected plants is very difficult to detect in the field until heading.
- Infected heads emerge earlier than normal heads.
- The entire inflorescence is commonly affected and appears as a mass of olive-black spores, initially covered by a thin gray membrane.
- Once the membrane ruptures, the head appears powdery.
- Spores are dislodged, leaving only the rachis intact.
- In some cases remnants of glumes and awns may be present on the exposed rachis.
- Smutted heads are shorter than healthy heads due to a reduction in the length of the rachis and peduncle.
- While infected heads are shorter, the rest of the plant is slightly taller than healthy plants.

2. Black or Stem Rust -*Puccinia graminis tritici*

Diagnostic Symptoms

On Wheat

- Stem rust occurs primarily on stems but can also be found on leaves, sheaths, glumes, awns and even seed.
- Symptoms begin as oval to elongate lesions that are generally reddish-brown in color.
- In the late stages of the disease, erumpent pustules produce numerous black sooty spores called telia are produced.

- For this reason stem rust is also known as 'black rust'.
- The telia are firmly attached to the plant tissue.
- Severe infestations with many stem lesions may weaken plant stems and result in lodging.

On Barberry

- Pycnia appear on barberry plants in the spring, usually in the upper leaf surfaces.
- They are often in small clusters and exude pycniospores in a sticky honeydew.
- Five to 10 days later, cup-shaped structures filled with orange-yellow, powdery aeciospores break through the lower leaf surface.
- The aecial cups are yellow and sometimes elongate to extend up to 5 mm from the leaf surface.

3. Brown or Leaf Rust - *Puccinia triticina (P. recondita)*

Diagnostic Symptoms

- Leaf rust is generally found on leaves but may also infect glumes and awns.
- Symptoms begin as small, circular to oval yellow spots on infected tissue of the upper leaf surface.
- As the disease progresses, the spots develop into orange colored pustules which may be surrounded by a yellow halo .
- The pustules produce a large number of spores that are easily dislodged from the pustule resulting in an "orange dust" on the leaf surface or on clothes, hands and equipment.
- As the disease progresses, black spores may be produced resulting in a mixture of orange and black lesions on the same leaf.
- Tiny orange lesions may be present on seed heads, but these lesions do not develop into erumpent pustules.
- Yield loss often occurs.

4. Yellow or Stripe Rust -*Puccinia striiformis*

Diagnostic Symptoms

- Stripe rust is distinguished by the presence of light yellow, straight-sided pustules that occur in stripes on leaves and heads.
- These elongate pustules are narrow and vary in length.
- As the pustules mature, yellow-orange spores are produced.
- As the disease progresses, tissues around the pustules turn brown and dry resulting in a scorched appearance.
- The arrangement of pustules into stripes is an important distinguishing characteristic of this disease.

5. Karnal Bunt -*Neovossia indica*

Diagnostic Symptoms

- Symptoms of karnal bunt are often difficult to distinguish in the field owing to the fact that incidence of infected kernels on a given head is low.
- Symptoms are most readily detected on seed after harvest.
- The black sorus, containing dusty spores is evident on part of the seed, commonly occurring along the groove.
- Heavily infected seed is fragile and the pericarp ruptures easily.
- The foul, fishy odor associated with karnal bunt.
- The odor is caused by the production of trimethylamine by the pathogen.
- Seed that is not extensively infected may germinate and produce healthy plants.

6. Flag Smut -*Urocystis tritici*

Diagnostic Symptoms

- The symptoms can be seen on stem, culm and leaves from late seedling stage to maturity.
- The seedling infection leads to twisting and drooping of leaves followed by withering.
- Grey to grayish black sori occurs on leaf blade and sheath.
- The sorus contains black powdery mass of spores.

7. Bunt or Stinking Smut -*Tilletia caries / T.foetida*

Diagnostic Symptoms

- In India disease occurs only in Northern hills, where wheat is grown.
- The diseased plants mature earlier and all the spikelets are affected.
- The pathogen attacks 8-10 days old seedling and become systemic and grows along the tip of shoot.
- At the time of flowering, hyphae concentrate in the inflorescence and spikelets and transforming the ovary into smut sorus of dark green color with masses of chlamydospores.

8. Powdery Mildew -*Blumeria graminis* f. sp. *tritici*

Diagnostic Symptoms

- Characterized by white, cottony patches of mycelium and conidia on the surface of the plant.
- They can occur on all aerial parts of the plant including stems and heads, but are most conspicuous on the upper surfaces of lower leaves.

- The white colonies later turn dull gray-brown.
- Severe infections can cause stunting.
- Heads on the later, shorter tillers can become heavily diseased because they remain lower in the wheat canopy where humidity is high.
- As the growing season progresses, sexual fruiting structures known as cleistothecia appear as distinct brown-black dots within aging colonies on maturing plants.
- When severe, individual patches often merge and cover large areas of the stem, leaf surface, or head.
- Leaf tissue on the opposite side of the mildew pustules becomes yellow, later turning tan or brown.

9. Leaf Blight -*Alternaria triticina*

Diagnostic Symptoms

- The disease appears when wheat plants are 7-8 weeks old and becomes severe when the crop is mature.
- Infection is first evident as small, oval, discoloured lesions irregularly scattered on the leaves.
- As the lesions enlarge they become dark brown to grey and irregular in shape.
- Some are surrounded by a bright-yellow marginal zone.
- The lesions vary in size, reaching a diameter of 1 cm or more.
- As the disease progresses, several lesions coalesce to cover large areas, resulting in the death of the entire leaf.
- In some cases the leaf starts drying up from the tip, prematurely, when lesions appear.
- The lowermost leaves are the first to show the signs of infection; the fungus gradually spreads to the upper leaves.
- In severe cases, similar symptoms are produced on the leaf sheath and stem, as well as the awns and glumes if spikes are infected at the pre-anthesis stage.
- If the spike is infected this early, seeds do not form.
- Infection at the dough stage of seed development results in glume infection, ear infection and seed infection.
- Heavily infected fields present a burnt appearance.

Crop stage wise IDM activities in Wheat		
Crop stage	Diseases	Step wise IDM practices
Wheat Off season/ pre-sowing	Soil and seed borne pathogens, Nematodes,	• Deep ploughing of fields during summer to control nematodes population, to popagules of soil borne pathogens. • Soil solarisation. • Timely sowing should be done. • Field sanitation, rogueing. • Destroy the alternate host plants. • Crop rotation with non-cereals. • Adopt ecological engineering by growing the attractant, repellent, and trap crops around the field bunds. • Apply well rotten farm yard manure only to discourage pathogen infestation. • Avoid late sowing of crops. • For nematode: Non host crops of gram, mustard, cumin, carrots, onion are suggested for 3 years. • For others follow common cultural practices. • Chemical control: For nematode: Carbofuran 3% CG @ 26640 g/acre.
Sowing/Seedling	For Loose smut:	• The seed is soaked in cold water during hot summer months in the morning hours and kept in hot sun from 8 am -12 noons and then dried in the afternoon. This kills the fungus inside the seed and provides a good disease measure without use of fungicides. However, precautions to be taken so that there is no damage to the viability of seeds. • Use resistant/tolarent varieties.
	For seed gall nematode	• Use certified seed resistance varieties only. • Clean seed by sieving or by using 2% salt water floatation to remove galls and prevent ear cockle diseases. • Use the tolerant varieties such as C-306 for brown mite. • Dry cleaning: Galls can be separated by coarse sieve from thehealthy seeds. • Winnowing or fanning • Brine floatation: 2% salt solution in place of plain water removes almost 100 % galls. Chemical Control: • For nematode: Carbofuran 3% CG @ 26640 g/acre. • For loose smut; Carboxin 75% WP @ 2 -2.5 g/Kg seeds or Tebuconazole 2% DS @ 0.2g/K seed or Carboxin 37.5% + Thiram 37.5% DS @ 3.0 g/Kg seed. • For flag smut: Carboxin 75% WP@2 -2.5 g/ Kg seed or Tebuconazole 2% DS@0.2g/Kg seed • For bunt: Carboxin 75% WP@ 2 -2.5 g/ Kg seed.

Vegetative/Ear head stage	Leaf rust, Stem rust and Yellow rust.	Cultural control: • Mixed cropping and crop rotation 0.2 g/Kg seed. • Avoid excess "N". Chemical control: • Spray Propiconazole 25% EC @ 200 ml in 200 l of water/acre or Tebuconazole 25% EC @ 200 ml in 200 l of water/acre or Thiophanate Methyl 70% WP@ 286 g in 300-400 l of water/acre.
	Powdery mildew	Cultural control: • The disease severity is more in some pockets and most of the present varieties do not have adequate resistance. Chemical control: • Spray Triadimefon 25% WP @ 200 g in 300 l of water/acre.
	Foliar blight, Seedling blight, Leaf spot, Leaf blight	Cultural control • Only use certified seed /resistance varieties. • Timely sowing seed, & crop rotation. • Plantation of tall plant crop as a barrier for air borne disease. Chemical control: • Spray Thiophanate Methyl 70% WP @ 1 g/L of water or Mancozeb +Carbendazim@ 2g/L water.
	Kernal bunt	Cultural control: • Low-lying areas of the field accumulate water and are more prone to KB. • Effective land leveling and drainage can reduce disease incidence. • Decrease seed rate during sowing. • Increase row spacing during sowing. • Delayed sowing. • Avoiding irrigation during the period of awn emergence and end of flowering may hinder disease development. • Avoid lodging by using balance dose of nitrogen and potash. • Plastic mulching or solarization reduces the chance of teliospore germination. Burn the stubble after harvesting. • Crop rotation with non-host crop. **Chemical control:** • Spray Propiconazole 25% EC@ 200 ml in 300 l of water/acre or Bitertanol25% WP@ 896 g in 300 l of water/acre.

	Loose smut, Hill bunt and Head scab, Flag smut	• For Loose smut: • Cultural Control • In the standing crop, the plants showing yellowing owing of the boot leaf tip normally are the ones which will give smutted ear heads on emergence. Uproot such plants before ear emergence to reduce the infestation of healthy seeds at later stage. Use disease free seeds in the healthy field. For seed production, disease free field/areas to be identified for having crop without considerable inoculum load.
		• Chemical control: • For Flag smut: Carboxin 75% WP@2 -2.5 gm/ Kg seed or Tebuconazole 2%• DS@0.2 g/Kg seed. • For Bunt: Carboxin 75% WP@ 2 -2.5 gm/ Kg seed. Triadimefon 25% WP @ 200 g in 300 l of water/acre. • For Loose smut: Same as pre-sowing stage.

19.3 IDM in Pearl Millet

Sl.No	Major Diseases	Causal Organism
1	Downy mildew	*Sclerospora graminicola*
2	Smut or Grain smut	*Tolyposporium penicillariae*
3	Rust	*Puccinia pennisetti*
4	Ergot or Sugary	*Claviceps fusiformis*

1. Downy Mildew (Green Ear)-*Sclerospora graminicola*

Diagnostic Symptoms

- Symptoms appear on leaves and inflorescence.
- The initial symptoms appear in seedlings at three to four leaf stages.
- The affected leaves show patches of light green to light yellow colour on the upper surface and the corresponding lower surface bears white downy growth of the fungus consisting of sporangiophores and sporangia.
- The yellow discolouration often turns to streaks along veins.
- As a result of infection young plants dry and die ultimately.
- The inflorescence of infected adult plants gets completely or partially malformed with florets converted into leafy structures, giving the typical symptom of **green ear**.

2. Smut or Grain Smut-*Tolyposporium penicillariae*

Diagnostic Symptoms

- The disease is observed on ear heads.
- The pathogen infects few florets and transforms them into sori containing smut spores.
- The sori are larger than normal healthy grains and when the sori mature they become dark brown releasing millions of black smut spore balls.
- The smut sori are formed in place of grains.
- Sori are oval , bigger than seeds and project beyond the glumes.

3. Ergot or Sugary - *Claviceps fusiformis*

Diagnostic Symptoms

- Exudation of small droplets of light pinkish or brownish honey dew from the infected spikelets.
- Under severe infection many such spikelets exude plenty of honey dew which trickles along the earhead.
- This attracts several insects.
- In the later stages, the infected ovary turns into small dark brown sclerotium which projects out of the spikelet.

4. Rust -*Puccinia pennisetti*

Diagnostic Symptoms

- Initial symptoms appear mostly on the distal half of the lamina.
- The leaf soon becomes covered by uredosori which appear more on the upper surface.
- The pustules may be formed on leaf sheath, stem and on peduncles.
- Later, telial formation takes place on leaf blade, leaf sheath and stem.
- While brownish uredia are exposed at maturity, the black telia remain covered by the epidermis for a longer duration.

Crop stage wise IDM activities in Pearl Millet		
Crop stage	Diseases	Step wise IDM practices
Pre – sowing/ sowing	Soil borne pathogens, nematodes	• Deep ploughing and soil solarisation to expose propagules of soil borne pathogens. • Timely sowing should be done. • Field sanitation, rogueing. • Destroy the alternate host plants. • Soil test based application of manures and fertilizers. • Adoption of crop rotation. • Sowing of healthy, disease free and certified seeds. • Uproot and burn infected plants early enough to avoid spread of the disease. • Avoid high plant populations
	Downy mildew, Smut and Nematodes	• Use tolerant/resistant varieties e.g. MH 1192,ICMH 451,Pusa 23, MBH 110, PHB 57, WC-C 75, ICTP 8203 and GHB 67 • Plant in a row of 15 inches to 24 inches. Seed may be placed about 6 inches apart within the row. • The seed should be planted shallow, about half inch deep . • Maintain good fertility levels, apply adequate organic manure
		• Apply neem cake @ 80 Kg/acre for nematode control. • Spray with fungicides metalaxyl 8%+ mancozeb 64%WP@ 800g in 200 l of water/acre for downy mildew. • Seed dressing with fungicides metalaxyl-M 31.8% ES@ 2.0 ml/Kg seed for downy mildew.
	Ergot	• Dipping the seeds in 10% NaCl salt solution for 10 minute. • The crop should be sown as early as possible during June-July with the onset of monsoon. • Use of resistant cultivars. • Eradicate the weeds like *Cenchrus ciliaris* and *Panicum antidotale* from around pearl millet fields.

	Downy mildew	• Roguing and gap filling, deep ploughing and soil solarisation. • Avoidance of monoculture. • Avoidance of low lying fields and water log. • Fungicide metalaxyl-M 31.8% ES used for seed treatment 2.0 ml/Kg seed. • Spray metalaxyl 8%+ mancozeb 64% WP@ 800g/acre in 200 l of water.
Vegetative Stage	Downy mildew	• As mentioned above in the sowing stage.
Flowering heading	Rust	• Follow the common cultural and mechanical practices. • Some fungal species controls rust disease such as *Aspergillus globosum*, *Chaetomium globosum* and *Trichoderma koningii.*
	Smut	• Avoid rationing. • Intercropping of mungbean with pearl millet.

19.4 IDM in Red Gram

Sl.No	Major Diseases	Causal Organism
1	Wilt	*Fusarium udum*
	Phytophthora blight	*Phytophthora drechsleri* f sp. *cajani*
2	Dry root rot	*Macrophomina phaseolina*
3	Powdery mildew	*Leveillula taurica*
4	Leaf spot	*Cercospora indica*
5	Alternaria blight	*A. alternata* and *A. tenuissima*
6	Sterility mosaic	*Pigeonpea sterility mosaic virus*
7	Yellow mosaic	*Mung bean yellow mosaic virus*

1. Wilt - *Fusarium udum*

Diagnostic Symptoms

- Patches of dead plants in the field when the crop is in flowering or podding stage are the first indication of wilt.
- The most characteristic symptom is a purple band extending upwards from the base of the main stem.
- Partial wilting of the plant is a definite indication of Fusarium wilt, and distinguishes this disease from termite damage, drought, and Phytophthora blight that all kill the whole plant.
- Partial wilting is associated with lateral root infection, while total wilt is due to tap root infection.
- The other characteristic symptom of wilt is browning of the stem tissue in the region of the purple band and browning or blackening of the xylem, visible when the main stem or primary branches are split open.
- Sometimes, branches (especially lower ones) dry, even if there is no band on the main stem.
- These branches have die-back symptoms with a purple band extending from tip downwards, and intensive internal xylem blackening.
- When young plants (1-2 months old) die from wilt, they may not show the purple band symptom, but have obvious internal browning and blackening.
- Plants infected by *F. udum* also exhibit a series of leaf symptoms before they die, including loss of leaf turgidity, interveinal clearing, and chlorosis to bright yellow.

2. Phytophthora Blight -*Phytophthora drechsleri* f sp. *cajani*

Diagnostic Symptoms

- At first, purple to dark brown necrotic lesions girdle the basal portion of the stem and later may occur an aerial parts.
- Initially lesions are small and smooth, later enlarging and slightly depressed.

- Infected tissues become soft and whole plant dies.
- Infection is mostly confined to basal portions of the stem in grown up plants
- The infected bark becomes brown and the tissue softens causing the plant to collapse.
- In leaf, localized yellowing starts from the tip and margin and progressively extends towards the mid-rib.
- The centre of the spots later turns brown and hard.
- The spots increase in size and cover a major portion of the lamina, leading to drying.

The gross symptoms of this disease resemble with wilt owing to which it has probably been mistaken for wilt disease in the past. However, both can be differentiated as:

- The leaves of plants affected by wilt turn yellow before drying while those of blight are light green with upward rolling followed by rapid drying.
- Leaves in case of wilt remain attached to plant while they shed in case of blight.
- Frequent blackening of xylem tissues in wilt and not in blight.

3. Dry Root Rot -*Macrophomina phaseolina*

Diagnostic Symptoms

- Infected seedlings show reddish brown discoloration at collar region.
- The lower leaves show yellowing, drooping and premature defoliation.
- The bark near the collar region shows shredding.
- The discolored area later turns to black and sudden death of the plants occurs in patches.
- The plant can be easily pulled off leaving dark rotten root in the ground.
- Minute dark sclerotia are seen in the shredded bark and root tissues.
- Huge number of brown dots seen on the stem portion represents the pycnidial stage of the fungus.

4. Alternaria Blight-*A. alternata* (Fr.) Keissler and *A. tenuissima* (Kauze ex Persoon)

Diagnostic Symptoms

- The symptoms appear on all aerial parts of the plant.
- Symptoms on leaves are small, circular, necrotic spots that develop quickly, forming typical concentric rings .Later, these spots coalesce and cause blighting of leaves.
- The spots are initially light brown and later turn dark brown.
- On stems, spots are sunken, with concentric rings.
- In severe infection, defoliation and drying of infected leaves, branches and flower buds is observed.

5. Leaf Spot -*Cercospora indica*

Diagnostic Symptoms

- First appear as small circular to irregular necrotic spots or lesions usually on older leaves.
- The spots later become dark brown and the infected portions drop off leaving shot hole.
- Irregular necrotic blotches develop when several spots join together and premature defoliation occurs.
- Black lesions develop on petioles and stem in severe cases.

6. Sterility Mosaic -*Pigeonpea sterility mosaic virus*

Diagnostic Symptoms

- SMD is often referred to as "green plague" as the affected plants are green with excessive vegetative growth but with no flowers or pods.
- SMD affected plants show characteristic mosaic symptoms that initially appear as vein clearing on leaves.
- The leaves are small and show a light and dark green mosaic pattern.
- In the field, the disease can be easily identified from a distance as patches of bushy, pale green plants without flowers or pods

7. Yellow Mosaic-*Mung bean yellow mosaic virus*

Diagnostic Symptoms

- Affected plants are conspicuous in the field, because of the green and golden yellow mosaic mottle symptoms on their leaves .
- Sometimes the affected parts of the leaves become necrotic.
- Diseased plants are usually scattered in the field, and may produce fewer pods than normal, especially when infected early.
- Off-season and isolated sowings suffer more from the disease than does the main-season crop.

Crop stage wise IDM activities in Pigeonpea		
Crop stage	Diseases	Step wise IDM practices
Off season/ pre-sowing	Soil and seed borne pathogens, Nematodes,	• Deep ploughing of fi elds during summer to control nematodes. • Three summer ploughings at 10 days interval reduce soil borne pathogens. • Soil solarization: Cover the beds with polythene sheet of 45 gauge (0.45 mm) thickness for three weeks before sowing for soil solarization which will help in reducing the soil borne pathogens. • Use resistant/tolerant varieties. • Select seeds from disease free fields. • Grow pigeon pea intercropped or mixed with cereal crops like sorghum. • Use certified and weed seed free seeds.
Sowing/ Seedling/ Vegetative stage /Flowering /pod formation stage	Wilt, Stem blight, Dry root rot	• Select a field with no previous record of wilt for at least past 3 years. • Uproot the wilted plant and use them as firewood or destroy them. • Avoid sowing redgram in fields with low-lying patches that are prone to water logging. • Treat seed with *Trichoderma viride* 1% WP@ 8 g/Kg seed and @ 200 g/acre for soil treatment (wilt & dry root rot). • Treat seed with Carboxin 37.5% + thiram 37.5% DS @ 4 g/Kg seed and 200 g/acre for soil treatment (wilt, stem blight and dry root rot). • Spray Thiophanate methyl 70% WP @ 0.1% (wilt). • Collect and destroy crop debris. • Judicious use of fertilizers.
		• Provide irrigation at critical stages of the crop. • Avoid water logging. • Avoid any stress to the crop as much as possible. • Collect and destroy disease infected and infested plant parts.
	Pigeon pea sterility mosaic (PSM), Mung bean yellow disease (MBYD)	• Follow the common cultural, mechanical and biological practices. • The spacing between the lines should be maintained at 30 to 40 cm. • Destroy sources of sterility mosaic inoculum. • Use yellow sticky traps for the control of whitefly insect vector of MBYD.

19.5 IDM in Bengal gram

Sl.No	Major Diseases	Causal Organism
1	Wilt	*Fusarium oxysporum* f.sp. *ciceris*
2	Rust	*Uromyces ciceris-arietini*
3	Ascochyta blight	*Ascochyta rabiei*
4	Collar rot	*Sclerotium rolfsii*
5	Dry root rot	*Rhizoctonia bataticola*
6	Wet root rot	*Rhizoctonia solani*
7	Botrytis gray mold	*Boirytis cinerea*
8	Alternaria blight	*Alternaria alternata* (Fr.) Keissl. and *Alternaria tenuis*
8	Anthracnose	*Colletotrichum dematium*

1.Wilt - *Fusarium oxysporum* f.sp. *ciceris*

Diagnostic Symptoms

- Chickpea foliage develops a greyish-green chlorosis, typically affecting lower leaves first and extending up the plant.
- Leaves eventually take on a dull-yellow colour, wilt and the plant collapses and dies.
- Adult plants wilt, with their petioles and rachises drooping.
- In some cases there may be leaf vein clearing before wilt begins.
- Internally, the xylem tissues stain dark brown to almost black.
- Wilting may initially affect only one side of the plant.

2. Rust -*Uromyces ciceris-arietini*

Diagnostic Symptoms

- Small oval, cinnamon brown, powdery lesions appear on both the surface, especially more on lower surface or leaf.
- The lesions, which are uredosori, cover the entire leaf surface.
- Dark teliosori appear on the leaves in the late season.
- The rust pustules may appear on petioles, stems and pods.
- Severely infected plants may dry up prematurely.

3. Ascochyta Blight - *Ascochyta rabiei*

Diagnostic Symptoms

- All above ground parts of the plant are infected.
- Round or elongated lesions, bearing irregularly depressed brown spot and surrounded by a brownish red margin on leaf.
- Similar spots may appear on the stem and pods.

- The spots on the stem and pods have pycnidia arranged in concentric circles as minute block dots.
- When the lesions girdle the stem, the portion above the point of attack rapidly dies.
- If the main stem is girdles at the collar region, the whole plant dies.

4. Collar Rot- *Sclerotium rolfsii*

Diagnostic Symptoms

- The disease comes in the early stages. (up to six weeks from sowing).
- Drying plants whose foliage turns slightly yellow before death, scattered in the field..
- The joint of stem and root turns soft slightly contracts and begins to decay.
- Infected parts turn brown white.
- Black dots, like mustard in shape known as sclerotia are seen appearing on the white infected plant parts.

5. Dry Root Rot -*Rhizoctonia bataticola*

Diagnostic Symptoms

- Dry root rot manifests symptoms from flowering to podding growth stage.
- Drooping of petioles and leaflets are the characteristic symptoms.
- Leaves and stems of affected plants becomes straw colored.
- When uprooted, the lower portion of the tap root remains in the soil.
- Dry root rot can be diagnosed by dark tap root and no lateral roots.
- Dark, minute sclerotia can be seen on the infected roots.

6. Wet Root Rot- *Rhizoctonia solani*

Diagnostic Symptoms

- Wet root rot is commonly seen at seedling stage.
- It can also occur at latter stages in irrigated condition.
- Affected seedling turn yellow with drooping petioles and leaflet.
- Seedling does not collapse.
- Diagnostic symptom is a sunken dark brown lesion above the collar region.
- Stem and root below the lesions rot and pinkish mycelial growth can be seen.
- Sclerotia not seen.

7. Botrytis Gray Mold- *Botrytis cinerea* pers. ex. Fr

Diagnostic Symptoms

- The disease is usually seen at flowering time when the crop canopy is fully developed.

- Lack of pod setting is the first indication of the disease.
- Under favorable conditions foliage shows clear symptoms and plants often die in patches.
- More severe on portions of the plant hidden under the canopy.
- Shed flowers and leaves, covered with the spore mass, can be seen on the ground under the plants.
- When humidity is very high, the symptoms appear on stems, leaves, flowers and pods as gray or dark brown lesions covered with moldy sporophores.
- Lesions on stem girdle the stem completely .
- Tender branches break off at the point where grey mold has caused rotting.
- Affected leaves and flowers turn into a rotting mass.
- Lesions on the pod are water soaked and irregular.
- Grayish white mycelium may be seen on the infected seeds.

7. Alternaria blight-*Alternaria alternata* (Fr.) Keissl.

Diagnostic Symptoms

- Water soaked, small, circular and purple lesions surrounded by chlorotic tissues on leaflets.
- Lesions later turn brown to dark brown.
- The infected flowers die.
- Circular, slightly sunken and irregularly scattered lesions on the pods.
- Affected pods turn dirty black.
- The pods contain shrivelled seeds.

Crop stage wise IDM activities in Chickpea		
Crop stage	Diseases	Step wise IDM practices
Off season/ pre-sowing/At sowing	Wilt/ Root rots	• Destruction of disease crop debris/ un-decomposed organic matter by deep tillage/ burn. • Timely sowing to avoid drought
	Ascochyta blight	• Destruction and burial of diseased crop debris by deep tillage. • Timely sowing to avoid drought. • Cultivation of resistant varieties (C235, GS43,CG558, Himachal channa1, Himachal channa 2, IPC 08-11, 23094, GNG 1581, GPF2, PBG5, Gaurav (H75-35),BG 267, Vardhan, Samrat).
	Botrytis grey mould	• Avoid late sowing and adopt wider spacing. • Cultivation of resistant variety (BG 276, GL90159, GL 9- 1071, GL92162, HK94-134, IPCK 2004- 29, ICC38, ICC 202, ICC1069). • Use disease free certified seed.
	Dry root rot/ Collar root rot	• Timely sowing to avoid drought. • Mild irrigation at the time of disease incidence under stress condition to minimize the soil temp. • Cultivation of resistant variety (JSC 37, JG 25174, CSJ 556, MPJG 89- 1155, MPJG 89-9023, CSJ 592, Rajas, JS 2000-07, ICCC 32, GL769).
	Nematode (Root knot, Reniform, Root lesion)	• Use of organic amendments including neem and castor cake @ 1 ton/ha 10 days before sowing in infested field and their combination with seed treatment with carbosulfan (25 DS) @ 3% a.i (w/w). • Seed treatment with *Trichoderma viride* each @ 10g/kg seed.
Seed & Seedling	Collar rot/ Dry root rot/ Botrytis grey mould, Ascochyta.	• Use Rhizobium culture @ 1pkt (200g) per ha for effective nodulation. • Thinning should be done a month after in case of dense plant population second spray
	Nematode	• Seed treatment with *Trichoderma viride* (effective strain) @ 10g/kg of seed.

19.6 IDM in Pea

Sl.No	Name of Disease	Causal Organism
1	Powdery mildew	*Erysiphe polygoni*
2	Downy mildew	*Peronospora pisi*
3	Rust	*Uromyces pisi (Pers.) Schrot*
4	Anthracnose	*Colletotrichum pisi*
5	Ascochyta blight	*Ascochyta pisi*
6	Septoria blotch	*Septoria pisi*
7	Bacterial blight	*Pseudomonas syringae* pv. *pisi* and *Pseudomonas syringae* pv. *syringae*

1. Powdery Mildew -*Erysiphe polygoni*

Diagnostic Symptoms

- Though the symptoms appear on every part of the pea plant, it is the leaves which show symptoms first.
- Infected plants are covered with a white powdery film, and severely infected foliage is blue-white in colour; tissue below these infected areas may turn purple.
- All aerial parts of the plant may become infected resulting in withering of the whole plant.
- Severe pod infection can cause a grey-brown discoloration of the seeds.
- These seeds have an objectionable flavour that lowers the quality of the grain.

2. Downy Mildew -*Peronospora pisi*

Diagnostic Symptoms

- This disease is most common soon after seedling emergence, but it may affect plants at any stage of growth especially during periods of moist, cool weather.
- Plants grown from infected seed are severely stunted and distorted, and have a sickly yellowish-green appearance.
- The undersides of the leaflets, in particular, are covered with a fluffy mouse-grey spore mass. Infected plants may turn yellow while producing an abundant source of spores, which cause secondary infections.
- Secondary infection results in the appearance of isolated greenish yellow to brown blotches on the upper surface of leaves while on the underside of the leaf, masses of mouse-grey colored spores are produced.
- The fungus usually affects the lowest leaves and then progresses up the plant, sometimes infecting flowers and pods.
- Infected pods are deformed and covered with yellow to brownish areas and superficial blistering.

3. Rust -*Uromyces pisi (Pers.) Schrot.*

Diagnostic Symptoms

- The disease appears usually at the beginning of flowering.
- Powdery orange-brown pustules (uredinia) containing uredospores are formed on both surface of leaves.
- They are small oval to round in shape and light brown in color. Severely infected leaves wither and fall off prematurely.
- Powdering dark brown telia containing teliospores appear at the end of summer. They are dark borwn and thinly distributed on the leaves.
- Aecia and pycnia are also produced occurring on the same host.
- Strongly affected leaves dry up and fall down, and beans remain undeveloped.

4. Anthracnose -*Colletotrichum pisi*

Diagnostic Symptoms

- The disease affects all above ground parts of plants.
- Irregularly-shaped grayish-smoky or brown spots are formed on leaves.
- Rounded or oval spots with dark brown limb and lighter center are formed on stalks.
- In the center orange-pink or reddish pads of sporiferous fungus are formed, having numerous setae.
- Conidia are colorless, unicellular, straight, or slightly bent, 10-20 x 3-4 microns in size.

Crop stage wise IDM activities in Pea		
Crop stage	Diseases	Step wise IDM practices
Pre-sowing/ Sowing	Soil and seed borne pathogens, Nematodes,	• Deep ploughing of fields during summer. Three summer ploughings at 10 days interval reduces soil borne pathogens. Timely sowing should be done. • Soil solarization: Cover the beds with transparent polythene sheet of 100 gauge thickness for three weeks before sowing for soil solarization which will help in reducing the soil-borne pests including weeds. • Field sanitation, rogueing. • Use resistant/tolerant varieties. • Avoid late sowing of the crop. • Destroy the alternate host plants. • Apply manures and fertilizers as per soil test recommendations. • Grow the attractant, repellent, and trap crops around the field bunds. • Crop rotation with non-host crops.

Vegetative stage	Powdery mildew	• Use resistant varieties. • Burn infected pea stubble soon after harvest where practicable. • Avoid sowing field pea crops adjacent to last season's stubble. • Control volunteer field peas which can harbour disease. • Adopt bower system. • Chemical control: Spray Fenarimol 12% EC @ 0.04% (40 ml/100 lts of water) as required depending on stage of crop. Second spray after 15 days of interval or sulphur 40% WP 2.26- 3.00 Kg in 300- 400 l of water per acre or Sulphur 80% WG @ 750 gm – 1.0 Kg in in 300- 400 l water per acre or Triadimefon 25% WP @ 0.1 % in 300 l water per acre. Second spray after 25 days of interval.
	Rust	• Destroy all diseased plant debris after harvest. • Follow suitable crop rotation with non-leguminous crops. • Mixed cropping. • Chemical control: sulphur 80% WP @ 1.252 Kg in 300-400 l water per acre or sulphur 85%DP @ 6 – 8 Kg per acre or triadimefon 25% WP @ 0.1 % in 300 l water per acre. Second spray after 25 days of interval.
	Downy mildew	• The diseased plants should be removed and burnt soon after detecting in the field. • Foliar spray with Mancozeb + Metalaxyl @ 2.5g/l, if required repeat after 25 days.
	Ascochyta blight	• Plantation of tall plant crop as a barrier for air borne inoculum.
	Root rot	• Keep wider spacing. • Maintain irrigation. • Follow common cultural practices.
	Fusarium wilt	• Follow common cultural practices.
Reproductive stages		• Same as in vegetative stage.

19.7 IDM in Black/Green Gram

Sl.No	Major Diseases	Causal Organism
1	Anthracnose	*Colletotrichum lindemuthianum*
2	Leaf spot	*Cercospora canescens*
3	Powdery mildew	*Erysiphe polygoni*
4	Rust	*Uromyces phaseoli*
5	Dry root rot	*Rhizoctonia bataticola*
6	Seed and Seedling rot	*Rhizoctonia solani, Macrophomina phaseolina, Pythium aphanidermatum, Sclerotium rolfsii*
7	Mungbean yellow mosaic	*Mungbean yellow mosaic virus*
8	Leaf curl / Necrosis	*Groundnut bud necrosis virus*

1. Anthracnose -*Colletotrichum lindemuthianum*

Diagnostic Symptoms

- The pathogen attacks all aerial parts of plants and at any stage of their growth.
- Initial symptoms are circular, black, sunken spots with dark center and bright red orange margins on leaves and pods.
- In severe infections, the affected parts wither off.
- Seedlings get blighted due to infection soon after seed germination.
- The infected pods have discolored seeds.

2.Cercospora Leaf Spot-*Cercospora canescens*

Diagnostic Symptoms

- Infected leaves show small, brown, water soaked, circular spots surrounded with yellowish halo.
- On older plants the leaflet infection is mostly on older leaves and may cause serious defoliation. The most striking symptoms are on the green fruit. Small water-soaked spots.
- Small water-soaked spots first appear which later become raised and enlarge until they are one-eighth to one-fourth inch in diameter.
- Centres of these lesions become irregular, light brown and slightly sunken with a rough, scabby surface.
- Ripe fruits are not susceptible to the disease. Surface of the seed becomes contaminated with the bacteria, remaining on the seed surface for some time.

3. Powdery Mildew -*Erysiphe polygoni*

Diagnostic Symptoms

- At first small, irregular powdery spots appear on the upper surface of the leaves, sometimes on both the surfaces.
- The disease becomes severe during flowering and pod development stage.

- The white powdery spots completely cover the leaves, petioles, stem and even the pods.
- The plant assumes greyish white appearance; leaves turn yellow and finally shed.
- Often pods are malformed and small with few ill-filled seeds.

4. Rust - *Uromyces phaseoli typica* (Syn: *U. appendiculatus*)

Diagnostic Symptoms

- The disease appears as circular reddish brown pustules which appear more commonly on the underside of the leaves, less abundant on pods and sparingly on stems.
- When leaves are severely infected, both the surfaces are fully covered by rust pustules.
- Shriveling followed by defoliation resulting in yield losses.

5. Dry Root Rot-*Rhizoctonia bataticola*

Diagnostic Symptoms

- The symptom starts initially with yellowing and drooping of the leaves.
- The leaves later fall off and the plant dies within week.
- Dark brown lesions are seen on the stem at ground level and bark shows shredding symptom. The affected plants can be easily pulled out leaving dried, rotten root portions in the ground.
- The rotten tissues of stem and root contain a large number of black minute sclerotia.

6. Mungbean Yellow Mosaic

Diagnostic Symptoms

- Initially mild scattered yellow spots appear on young leaves.
- The next trifoliate leaves emerging from the growing apex show irregular yellow and green patches alternating with each other.
- Spots gradually increase in size and ultimately some leaves turn completely yellow.
- Infected leaves also show necrotic symptoms.
- Diseased plants are stunted, mature late and produce very few flowers and pods.
- Pods of infected plants are reduced in size and turn yellow in colour.

7. Leaf Crinkle -*Urdbean leaf crinkle virus* (ULCV)

Diagnostic Symptoms

- Crinkling and curling of the tips of leaflets.
- Crinkling and rugosity in older leaves becomes severe and leaves thickened.

- Petioles as well as internodes are shortened.
- Infected plant gives a stunted and bushy appearance.
- Flowering is delayed.
- If inflorescence is formed, is malformed with small size flower buds and fails to open.

Crop stage wise IDM activities in Urd/Mung bean		
Crop stage	Diseases	Step wise IDM practices
Off season/ pre-sowing/At sowing	Soil borne pathogens Nematodes, Resting stage of pathogen	• Deep ploughing of fields during summer. • After summer ploughing field is left for solarization. • Timely sowing should be done. • Field sanitation, rogueing. • Destroy the alternate host plants. • Apply manures and fertilizers as per soil test recommendations. • Use tolerant/ resistant varieties. • Sow the ecological engineering plants. • Rotate the crop with a non host cereal crop, cucurbit, or cruciferous.
Vegetative / flowering stage	Anthracnose, Bacterial leaf blight, Cercospora leaf spot	• Early planting i.e. immediately after onset of monsoon. • Grow crop on bower system to avoid soil contact. • Maintain proper drainage in the field.
	Powdery mildew	• Bower system (maintain gapping) of cropping reduces the disease incidence. • Spray Penconazole 10% EC@ 20ml diluted in 200 l of water/acre.
	Rust	• Volunteer plants reduce the disease severity
	Root rot, Macrophomina blight	• Plant in well-draining soils. • Prepare seed beds to enhance rapid germination. • Proper irrigation is provided to prevent flooding and saturated soil condition. • Soil amendment with farm yard manure @ 5 tonnes/acre.
	Yellow mosaic virus. Leaf crinkle virus	• Collect and destroy crop debris. • Collect and destroy disease infected infected plant parts. • Avoid water logging. • Judicious use of fertilizers. • Avoid any stress to the crop as much as possible. • Avoid excessive use of nitrogenous fertilizers. • Rogueing and destroying the infested plants.

19.8 IDM in Rape Seed & Mustard

Sl.No	Major Diseases	Causal Organism
1	White rust	*Albugo candida*
2	Alternaria blight	*Alternaria brassicae, A. brassicicola*, and *A.raphani*
3	Downy mildew	*Peronospora parasitica*
4	Powdery mildew	*Erysiphe cruciferarum*
5	Sclerotinia stem rot	*Sclerotinia sclerotiorum*
6	Club root	*Plasmodiophora brassicae*
7	Bacterial blight/ Black rot	*Xanthomonas campestris* pv. *campestris*

1.White Rust-*Albugo candida*

Diagnostic Symptoms

- All the above ground parts may show infection.
- White rust pathogens create chlorotic (yellowed) lesions and sometimes galls on the upper leaf surface.
- There are corresponding white blister-like dispersal pustules of sporangia on the underside of the leaf.
- The branches and flower parts of mustard deformed.
- The pathogen stimulates hypertrophy and hyperplasia.
- The disease is sometimes called the cancer of rapeseed as one phase of this disease shows malformation of the young shoots and inflorescence.
- The flower and young fruits may also malformed.
- Such malformed pod lack seed development.

2.Alternaria Blight- *Alternaria brassicae, A. brassicicola*, and *A.raphani.*

Diagnostic Symptoms

- The disease attacks on the lower leaves as small circular brown necrotic spots which slowly increase in size.
- Many concentric spots coalesce to cover large patches showing blightening and defoliation in severe cases.
- Circular to linear, dark brown lesions also develop on stems and pods, which are elongated at later stage.
- Infected pods produce small, discolored and shriveled seeds.

3. Downy Mildew-*Peronospora parasitica,*

Diagnostic Symptoms

- Grayish white irregular necrotic patches develop on the lower surface of leaves.
- Later under favorable conditions brownish white fungal growth may also be seen on the spots.

- The most conspicuous and pronounced symptom is the infection of inflorescence causing hypertrophy of the peduncle of inflorescence and develop stag head structure.

4. Sclerotinia Stem Rot (White Mold) -*Sclerotinia sclerotiorum.*

Diagnostic Symptoms

- Initial symptoms appear as the plant canopy closes over rows during flowering and pod development.
- Lodged stems in contact with the soil develop watery lesions, with snowy white mycelium and black, irregularly shaped sclerotia become apparent as disease progresses.
- When the stem is completely girdled by such lesions, the plants wilt and die.
- When the crop is at seed stage, the plants tend to lodge, touching the siliquae to the soil level. Such plant show rotting of the siliquae with fungal growth along with the sclerotial, bodies just above the soil level.

5. Powdery Mildew-*Erysiphe cruciferarum*

Diagnostic Symptoms

- Symptoms appear as dirty white, circular, floury patches on either sides of the leaves.
- Under favorable environmental conditions, entire leaves, stems, floral parts and pods are affected.
- The whole leaf may be covered with powdery mass.

6. Bacterial Blight/ Black Rot-*Xanthomonas campestris pv. campestris*

Diagnostic Symptoms

- The leaf tissue turns yellow and chlorosis reach towards the centre of the leaf and form V shaped area with base of V towards the midrib.
- The veins show brown to black discoloration.
- Dark coloured streaks are formed on the stem from the ground level and gradually these streaks enlarge and girdle the stem.
- Stem become hollow due to internal rotting.
- Midrib cracking of lower leaves, browning of veins and withering is observed.
- In severe cases, the vasicular bundles of the stem also turn brown and the plant collapses.

Crop stage wise IDM activities in Rape Seed &Mustard		
Crop stage	Diseases	Step wise IDM practices
Off season/ pre-sowing/At sowing	Defoliators/soil borne pathogens	• Deep ploughing to expose the soil borne pathogens. • Prepare the level and well drained fi eld to reduce the incidence of Sclerotinia rot. • Destruction of plant debris. • For club rot management, soil amendment with lime (@ 1 Kg/m2) to raise soil pH to 7.2 or apply Neem cake @ 0.5 Kg/m2 .
Seedling	White rust/ Downy mildew	• Use certified seeds of resistant/tolerant variety. • Follow timely sowing of crop. • Adopt proper field sanitation. • Follow proper crop rotation. • Destruct crop debris particularly stag heads of previous year crop. • Avoid over irrigation or water stagnation. • Apply potash in recommended dose. • Treat the seeds with freshly prepared garlic bulb extract @ 2% (w/v). • Treat seed with Metalaxyl 35% WS @ 0.75- 1.0 Kg/100 Kg seed. • Spray Metalaxyl 8% + Mancozeb 64% WP @0.25% (white rust).
	Nematode	• Seed treatment with *Trichoderma viride* (effective strain) @ 10g/kg of seed.
Vegetative	Alternaria leaf spot	• Use certified/resistant/tolerant variety of seeds. • Adopt timely sowing between10-25 October. • Follow proper field sanitation. • Remove weeds particularly collateral host plants. • Apply recommended dose of potash to reduce disease incidence. • Foliar spray with Metalaxyl 8% + Mancozeb 64% WP @0.25%
	White rust and downy mildew	• Same as sowing stage.
	Bacterial blight	• Follow proper crop and fi eld sanitation. • Follow proper crop rotation.
	Powdery mildew	• Follow timely sowing of seeds. • Adopt proper fi eld sanitation. • Destruct crop infected crop residues. • Apply potash in recommended dose.
Flowering	Alternaria blight	• Same as vegetative stage.
	White rust, Downy mildew	• Same as vegetative stage.

	Club root	• Follow long term crop rotation. • Destroy all cruciferous weeds. • Follow timely crop sowing between 10-25 October. • Improve the drainage system.
	Sclerotinia stem rot	• Implement deep ploughing during summer. • Use certified seeds of resistant/tolerant varieties. • Follow timely sowing of crop. • Use proper field sanitation practices. • Follow crop rotation with non host crops like, rice and maize.
	Powdery mildew	• Same as vegetative stage

19.9 IDM in Sugarcane

Sl.No	Major Diseases	Causal Organism
1	Red rot	*Colletotrichum falcatum*
2	Smut	*Ustilago scitaminea*
2	Wilt	*Cephalosporium sacchari*
3	Gummosis	*Xanthomonas axonopodis* pv. *vasculorum*
4	Rust	*Puccinia erianthi*
5	Sett rot or Pineapple	*Ceratocystis paradoxa*
6	Red stripe	*Pseudomonas rubrilineans*
7	Mosaic	*Sugarcane mosaic potyvirus*
8	Grassy shoot	*Phytoplasma*
9	Ratoon stunting	*Clavibacter xyli* sub sp. *xyli*
10	Leaf Scald	*Xanthomonas albilineans* (Ashby)

1. Red Rot -*Colletotrichum falcatum*

Diagnostic Symptoms

- The first external symptom appears mostly on third or fourth leaf which withers away at the tips along the margins.
- Typical symptoms of red rot are observed in the internodes of a stalk by splitting it longitudinally.
- These include the reddening of the internal tissues which are usually elongated at right angles to the long axis of the stalk.
- The presence of cross-wise white patches are the important diagnostic character of the disease. The diseased cane also emits acidic-sour smell. As the disease advances, the stalk becomes hollow and covered with white mycelial growth.
- Later the rind shrinks longitudinally with minute black, velvety fruiting bodies protruding out of it.
- The pathogen also produces tiny reddish lesions on the upper surface of leaves with dark dots in the centre.
- The lesions are initially blood red with dark margins and later on with straw coloured centres. Often the infected leaves may break at the lesions and hang down, with large number of minute black dots.

2. Smut- *Ustilago scitaminea*

Diagnostic Symptoms

- Formation of characteristic whip-like, pencil-thick unbranched structures from the apices of affected stem.
- Each structure comprises a core of parenchyma and fibrovascular elements surrounded by vast numbers of chlamydospores, enclosed at first in a thin, silvery sheath.

- Later, when the membranous covering splits, the exposed chlamydospores resemble a thick layer of soot. They are then dispersed, mainly by wind.
- Smut is transmitted in two ways: by windborne spores gaining entry into standing cane through the buds; and by spores in the soil, or in irrigation water, entering planted setts.
- Infected buds may develop quickly into whips, or the mycelia may remain dormant within the buds to form a latent source of disease if the stems are used as a seed-cane.

1. Wilt - *Cephalosporium sacchari*

Diagnostic Symptoms

- The initial symptom of the disease is visible in the canes of 4-5 month age.
- The affected plants are stunted with yellowing and withering of crown leaves.
- The midribs of all leaves in a crown generally turn yellow, while the leaf lamina may remain green.
- The leaves dry up and stem develop hollowness in the core.
- The canes may wither in groups.
- The core shows the reddish discolouration with longitudinal red streaks passing from one internode to another.
- In severe cases, spindle shaped cavities tapering towards the nodes develop in each internode.
- The canes emit a disagreeable odour, with lot of mycelial threads of the fungus cover the cavity.

2. Rust -*Puccinia erianthi (Syn: P. melanocephala and P. kuehnii)*

Diagnostic Symptoms

- The earliest symptoms of common rust on the leaves are small, elongated yellowish spots which are visible on both the surfaces.
- These spots increase in size, mainly in length, and turn red-brown to brown in color. A narrow, pale yellow-green halo develops around the lesions.
- When the common rust is severe, numerous lesions occur on individual leaves giving them an overall brown or rusty appearance.
- These lesions coalesce to from large, irregular necrotic areas is usually result in premature death of the leaf. In such cases, the number of live leaves per plant can be seriously reduced, while in very susceptible varieties there may be fewer stalks per stool and reduced diameter and length of the stalks.

- Affected crops take on a distinctive rusty to brown color, as disease intensity builds up.
- The discoloration of these crops is readily seen from a distance.
- In some cases, bands of lesions may occur; resulting from intermittent heavy infection while the leaf is in the partially unrolled spindle.
- Rust can also cause wilting, some leaf tip death and accelaterated death of leaves.

5. Grassy Shoot - *Phytoplasma*

Diagnostic Symptoms

- The initial symptom appears nearly two months after planting.
- The disease is characterized by proliferation of vegetative buds from the base of the cane giving rise to crowded bunch of tillers bearing narrow leaves.
- Leaves become pale yellow to completely chlorotic, thin and narrow.
- The plants appear bushy and 'grass-like' due to reduction in the length of internodes premature and continuous tillering.
- The affected clumps are stunted with premature proliferation of auxillary buds.
- Cane formation rarely occurs in the affected clumps, if formed, thin with shorter internodes having aerial roots at the lower nodes.
- The buds on such canes usually papery and abnormally elongated.

6. Ratoon Stunting -*Clavibacter xyli* sub sp. *xyli* (*Rickettsia like organism - RLO)*

Diagnostic Symptoms

- Diseased clumps usually display stunted growth, reduced tillering, thin stalks with shortened internodes and yellowish foliage.
- Orange-red vascular bundles in shades of yellow at the nodes are seen in the infected canes.

Crop stage wise IDM activities in Sugarcane		
Crop stage	Diseases	Step wise IDM practices
Sowing	Soil & seed borne diseases	• Deep ploughing in summer and left undisturbed 20-25 days. • Cross ploughing of land followed by clod crushing and 1-2 harrowing. • Select tolerant / resistant varieties. • Select the seed cane from aerated steam treated nurseries. • Adopt paired row method of planting.
	Nematodes	• Deep ploughing, solarisation, fl ooding, crop rotation and apply organic manure. • Under wetland conditions, intercropping with sun hemp or marigold or daincha. • Apply pressmud at 6 t/acre or poultry manure @ 0.8 t/acre or neem cake 0.8 t/acre or poultry manure @ 0.4 t/acre before last ploughing. • Application of biocontrol agents like *Pochonia chlamydosporia, Paecilomyces lilacinus or Trichoderma viride* or *Pseudomonas fl uorescens* @ 4 Kg/acre at the time of planting mixed with moist FYM or cured pressmud and distributed uniformly helps in suppressing the plant parasitic nematodes.
Cane formation stage	Red rot, Smut, Grassy shoot, Wilt, Leaf scald, Red stripe, Mosaic. Rust and Pokkahboeng	• Use resistant or moderately resistant varieties. • Any sett showing reddening at the cut ends or at the nodal region should be discarded. • Healthy setts should be planted. Such setts must be produced from crop raised from heat treatment of seed canes in moist hot air at 54° C for 2.5 hour at 99% humidity. • Remove affected clump along with root system and burn. • Bunding of aff ected field should be done to avoid movement of rain or fl oodwater to healthy fields. • Ratooning of diseased crop should be avoided. • Diseased crop should be harvested as early as possible. • Crop rotation should be followed in affected fields.

19.10 IDM in Cotton

Sl.No	Major Diseases	Causal Organism
1	Wilt	*Fusarium oxysporum* f.sp. *vasinfectum*
2	Verticillium wilt	*Verticillium dahliae*
3	Para wilt/New wilt / Sudden Wilt	Physiological disorder
4	Root rot	*Rhizoctonia solani*
5	Anthracnose	*Colletotrichum capsici*
6	Grey or Areolate mildew	*Ramularia areola*
7	Boll rot	*Fusarium moniliforme, Colletotrichum capsici, A. niger, Rhizopus nigricans, Aspergillus flavus, Nematospora nagpuri* and *Botryodiplodia* sp.
8	Leaf blight	*Alternaria macrospora*
9	Bacterial blight	*Xanthomonas axonopodis* pv. *malvacearum*
10	Leaf curl	*Cotton leaf curl virus*

1.Wilt-*Fusarium oxysporum* f.sp. *vasinfectum*

Diagnostic Symptoms

- The disease affects the crop at all stages.

Seedling stage

- Cotyledons of the seedling turn yellow and then brown.
- The base of petiole shows brown ring, followed by wilting and drying of the seedlings.

Young and grown up plants

- Symptoms start from the older leaves at the base, followed by younger ones towards the top, finally involving the branches and the whole plant.
- Initial symptom is yellowing of edges of leaves and area around the veins i.e. discoloration starts from the margin and spreads towards the midrib.
- The leaves loose their turgidity, gradually turn brown, droop and finally drop off.
- The defoliation or wilting may be complete leaving the stem alone standing in the field.
- Sometimes partial wilting occurs; where in only one portion of the plant is affected, the other remaining free.
- Browning or blackening of vascular tissues is the other important symptom,
- Black streaks or stripes may be seen extending upwards to the branches and downwards to lateral roots.
- In severe cases, discolouration may extend throughout the plant starting from roots extending to stem, leaves and even bolls.
- In transverse section, discoloured ring is seen in the woody tissues of stem.

- The plants affected later in the season are stunted with fewer bolls which are very small and open before they mature.

2. Verticillium Wilt -*Verticillium dahliae*

Diagnostic Symptoms

- The first symptoms can be seen as bronzing of veins by interveinal chlorosis and yellowing of leaves.
- Lastly the leaves begin to dry, giving a scorched appearence.
- At this stage, the characteristic diagnostic feature is the drying of the leaf margins and areas between veins, which gives a "**Tiger stripe" or "Tiger claw**" appearance.
- The affected leaves fall off leaving the branches barren.
- Infected roots and stem, when split open, show a pinkish discolouration of the woody tissue which may taper off into longitudinal streaks in the upper parts and branches.
- The infected leaf also shows brown spots at the end of the petioles.
- The affected plants may bear a few smaller bolls with immature lint.
- Plants infected at early stages are severely stunted.

3. Para wilt/New wilt /Sudden Wilt

Diagnostic Symptoms

- The wilt may develop either slow or quick.
- The incidence is particularly high in plants with large canopy and heavy boll load.
- In the affected plants, leaves show wilt like drooping, become chlorotic and turn bronze or red followed by drying.
- Premature abscission of leaves and fruiting parts may occur.
- Leaves lose turgidity due to enhanced transpiration.
- Squares and young bolls are shed and immature bolls are forcefully opened.
- Wilted plants show development of anthocyanin pigment.
- Most of the wilted plants gradually recover and produce new flushes, however their contribution to yield is negligible.

Causes

- Higher demand for nutrients and moisture.
- Cultivation of susceptible varieties/hybrids.
- Prolonged dry spell with high temperature and sunlight followed by soil saturation due to heavy downpour or irrigation.
- Wilt incidence is high in heavy clayey and deep soils.
- Incidence is more in ill drained soils as compared to well drained soils.

4. Anthracnose - *Colletotrichum capsici*

Diagnostic Symptoms

- The pathogen infects the seedlings and produces small reddish circular spots on the cotyledons and primary leaves.
- The lesions develop on the collar region, stem may be girdled, causing seedling to wilt and die.
- In mature plants, the fungus attacks the stem, leading to stem splitting and shredding of bark.
- The most common symptom is boll spotting.
- Small water soaked, circular, reddish brown depressed spots appear on the bolls.
- The lint is stained to yellow or brown, becomes a solid brittle mass of fiber.
- The infected bolls cease to grow and burst and dry up prematurely.

Crop stage wise IDM activities in Cotton		
Crop stage	Diseases	Step wise IDM practices
Off season/ pre-sowing/At sowing	Soil and seed borne pathogens, Nematodes,	• Select tolerant/resistant cultivars. • Acid delinting treatment for seeds. • Seed treatment with Thiram 75% WS @ 2.5-3.0 gm/kg seeds. • Seed borne infection can be eliminated by soaking the seeds in 40 to 50 ppm solution of Streptomycin Sulphate 90% + Tetracycline Hydrochloride 10% SP for a period of two hours.
Early fruiting stage (50-80 days)	CLCuD	• Destroy affected plants (for Northern India).
	Parawilt	• Foliar application of 10ppm cobalt chloride on infected plants.
Peak flowering & fruiting stage (80-120 days)	Black arm.	• Spray recommended chemicals (Streptomycin Sulphate 90% + Tetracyline Hydrocloride 10% SP). Streptocycline 25-40 ppm to be sprayed thrice - Before flowering, after flowering and twenty days after second spray.
	Leaf reddening	• Foliar application of urea (1-2 %) with 15-20 ppm chlormequat chloride and 0.10 % citric acid, 2-3 times at weekly intervals.
	Parawilt	• Foliar application of 10 ppm cobalt chloride on infected plants.

19.11 IDM in Mango

Sl.No	Name of Disease	Causal organism
1	Anthracnose	*Colletotrichum gloeosporioides*
2	Powdery mildew	*Oidium mangiferae (Acrosporium mangiferae)*
3	Mango malformation	*Fusarium moniliforme* var. *subglutinans*
4	Stem end rot	*Botrydiplodia theobromae*
5	Red rust	*Cephaleurus mycoides*
6	Grey blight	*Pestalotia mangiferae*
7	Sooty mould	*Capnodium mangiferae*

Major diseases and their diagnostic symptoms

1. Anthracnose: *Colletotrichum gloeosporioides*

Diagnostic Symptoms

- Produces leaf spots, blossom blight, wither tip, twigs blight and fruit rot.
- Small blister like spots develop on the leaves and twigs. Young leaves wither and dry. Tender twigs wither and die back symptom appears.
- Affected branches ultimately dry up. Black spots appear on fruits.
- The fruit pulp becomes hard, crack and decay at ripening.
- Infected fruits drop.

2. Powdery mildew: *Oidium mangiferae (Acrosporum mangiferae)*

Diagnostic Symptoms

- The characteristic symptom of the disease is the white superficial powdery fungal growth on leaves, stalk of panicles, flowers and young fruits.
- Generally the infection begins from the tip of the inflorescence and spread downwards.
- The security of the disease reduces both number and size of the fruit.
- The affected flowers and fruits drop pre-maturely reducing the crop load considerably or might even prevent the fruit set.

3. Mango malformation : *Fusarium moliliforme* var. *subglutinans*

Diagnostic Symptoms

- Two types of symptoms: floral malformation and vegetative malformation.
- In vegetative malformation, excessive vegetative branches of limited growth in seedlings. They are swollen with short internodes forming bunches of various size and the top of the seedlings shows bunchy top appearance.
- In malformation of inflorescens, shows variation in the panicle. Malformed head dries up in black mass and persist for long time.

- Secondary branches are transformed into number of small leaves giving a witches broome appearance.

4. Red-rust: *Cephaleuros virescens*

Diagnostic Symptoms

- Algae attacks foliage and young twigs.
- Rusty spots appear on leaves, initially as circular, slightly elevated coalesce to form irregular spots.
- The spores mature fall off and leave cream to white valvet texture on the surface of the leaves.

5. Grey Blight : *Pestalotia mangiferae*

Diagnostic Symptoms

- Brown spots develop on the margin and at the tip of the leaf lamina. They increase in size and become dark brown. Black dots appear on the spots which are acervuli of the fungus.
- Survive on mango leaves for over a year. Spreads through wind borne conidia.
- Heavy infection is noticed during the monsoon when the temperature is 20-25 °C and high humidity.

6. Sooty mould : *Capnodium mangiferae*

Diagnostic Symptoms

- The disease is characterized by the presence of a black velvety thin membraneous covering on the leaf surface.
- In severe cases , the tree appears black due to heavy infestation of moulds on entire surface of leaves and twigs which affect the photosynthetic activity.
- Because of the production of masses of black spores, which adhere to the leaf surface due to sticky honey dew the foliage appears black, ugly and hence the name 'sooty mould' is given.
- During flowering time, if the fungus infects the blossome, fruit setting is affected and sometimes even small fruits may fall.

7. Bacterial leaf spot: *Pseudomonas mangiferae- indicae*

Diagnostic Symptoms

- Symptoms are seen on leaves and fruits.
- On the leaves initially slightly water soaked yellowish, translucent irregular spots are formed towards leaf tip which enlarge soon and become dark brown with a yellow halo.
- These dark spots are limited by veins and become angular resulting in cankerous raised lesions.

- Spots appear all over the lamina.
- Under high humid conditions these spots fuse, leaves turn yellow and drop down prematurely.
- Longitudinal cracks develop on petioles.
- On green twigs, dark lesions of infection spread to inflorescence stalks.
- When fruits are attacked, water soaked lesion develop and turn dark brown to black.
- The affected fruits become yellow with deep cracks severely affected fruits are shed prematurely.

Crop stage wise IDM activities in Mango		
Crop stage	Diseases	Step wise IDM practices
Pre planting/ Planting	Soil borne pathogens, Nematodes	• Destroy the alternate host plants. • Sow the ecological engineering plants. • Rogue out diseased seedling. • Use resistant/tolerant varieties. • Destroy the alternate host plants. • Well decomposed farm yard manure coupled with *Trichoderma viride/harzianum* should be used. • Nursery beds should be raised. • Nursery beds should be fumigated with 4% formalin. • Deep summer ploughing of field reduces the incidence of soil-borne pathogens. • Medium size nuts (7-9 gm) may be selected to get vigorously growing seedlings.
		• Seed nuts should be soaked over night in water before sowing. • Sow the soaked nuts in the polythene bags filled with potting mixture. • Irrigate the orchards as and when required. • Provide proper shade, irrigation & drainage.
Vegetative stage	Powdery mildew	• Follow common cultural, mechanical and biological practices. • Spraying at full bloom needs to be avoided. • Prune diseased leaves and malformed panicles harbouring the pathogen to reduce primary inoculum load. • Chemical control: Azoxystrobin 23% SC @ 100 ml (0.1%)/100 l of water depending on the size of the tree canopy or Hexaconazole 5% EC@ 0.1%(100ml/100 l) depending on the size of tree or Penconazole 10% EC@50ml/100Lt. water or Sulphur 55.16 % SC@ 0.30%or300 ml/100Lt. water or Triadimefon 25% WP@ 0.040- 0.100% ,10-15 l depending on the size of tree

	Anthracnose	• Follow common cultural, mechanical and biological practices. • Cultural Control: Diseased leaves, twigs, gall midge infected leaves and fruits, should be collected and burnt. • Covering the fruits on tree, 15 days prior to harvest with news or brown paper bags. • Chemical Control: Azoxystrobin 23% SC@ 100 ml (0.1%)/100 l of water depending on the size of the tree canopy. Copper oxy-chloride 50% WG@0.24%or 240g/100lwater as required depending upon PP equipment
	Dieback	• Follow common cultural, mechanical and biological practices. • Scion wood selected for propagation should be free from infection. • Every care should be taken to prevent introduction of disease in newly planted orchards. • Any infected portion should immediately be pruned, followed by spraying/ pasting of copper oxy-chloride or pasting with cow dung at the cut ends. • Pruning should be done in such a way that some healthy portion is also removed, to ensure complete eradication of pathogen (3 "below the infection site)
	Bacterial canker	• Follow common cultural, mechanical and biological practices. • Regular inspection of orchards, sanitation and seedling certification are recommended as preventive measures. • Mango stones for raising seedlings (root stock) should always be taken from healthy fruits. • Use of wind-breaks helps in reducing brushing/ wounding and thus reduces chance of infection.
	Red rust	• Follow common cultural, mechanical and biological practices . • If vigour of plant is maintained by balanced nutrients, the disease is less. • As the disease starts on the onset of rain, it is desired to spray fungicide copper oxy-chloride twice during the month of July/ August at 15 days intervals.
Reproductive	Powdery mildews, Anthracnose, Dieback, Bacterial canker, Red rust, Phoma blight	• Same as vegetative stage.

	Mango malformation	• The floral malformed panicles/ vegetative malformed shoots should be pruned and burnt which reduces the incidence of malformation. • Application of NAA (200 ppm) in the first week of October (Before bud differentiation stages) followed by deblossoming in the late December or January reduces the incidence of malformation.
Maturation	Sooty mould, Anthracnose, Bacterial canker	• Same as vegetative stage
	Anthracnose, Stem end rot, Aspergillus rot	• Hot water treatment at 52 °C for 4-5min. • Fruits should be sprayed with the mixture of bio-inoculants. • Postharvest dip treatment of fruits with botanical fungicides could also control the diseases during storage.

19.12 IDM in Banana

Sl.No	Name of Disease	Causal Organism
1	Panama	*Fusarium oxysporum* f. sp. *cubense*
2	Moko	*Pseudomonas solanacearum / Burkholderia solanacearum*
3	Sigatoka	*Mycosphaerella gloeosporioides*
4	Anthracnose	*Gloeosporium gloeosporioides*
5	Bunchy top	*Banana bunchy top virus*

Major Diseases and their Diagnostic Systems

1. Panama wilt: *Fusarium oxysporum* f. sp *cubense*

Diagnostic Symptoms

- Symptoms are most clear on the plant s that are at least five month old.
- Sudden wilting of the plant or individual leaves is a characteristic symptom of the disease.
- Yellowing of the lower most leaves starting from margin to midrib of the leaves.
- Yellowing extends upwards and finally heart leaf alone remains green for some time and it is also affected.
- The leaves break near the base and hang down around pseudostem.
- Discolored vascular strands varying from light yellow to dark brown are the distinguishing internal symptoms.
- Usually the discoloration manifests first in the outer or oldest leaf sheath and extends upto the pseudostem.

2. Moko: *Pseudomonas solanacearum / Burkholderia solanacearum*

Diagnostic Symptoms

- Symptoms start on rapidly growing young plants.
- The youngest three to four leaves turn pale green or yellow and collapse near the junction of lamina and petiole.
- Characteristic discoloration of vascular strands, wilting and blackening ofsuckers.
- Vascular discolouration (pale yellow to dark brown or bluish black) is concentrated near the centre of the pseudostem, becoming less apparent on the periphery.
- Greyish brown bacterial ooze is seen when the pseudostem of affected plant is cut transversely.
- A firm brown dry rot is found within fruits of infected plants (characteristic symptom).

3. Sigatoka : *Mycosphaerella musicola (Cercospora musae)*

Diagnostic Symptoms

- Early symptoms appear on the young leaves.
- Small spindle shaped spots on foliage with greyish centre and yellowish halo running parallel to veins.
- Spots are mostly seen along the edge of the leaf with defined margin and possess dark brown to black margin. Spots coalesce and whole leaf blade dries up.
- On the upper surface of the spots, fructifications of the fungus appear as black specks.
- Unevenly and individual bananas appear undersized and their flesh develops a buff pinkish colour, and store poorly.

4. Anthracnose : *Gloeosporium gloeosporioides*

Diagnostic Symptoms

- The skin at the distal ends of the fingers turn black, shrivels.
- The fungus produces masses of conidia which form a pinkish coat.
- The entire fruit and bunch is affected in severe cases. Sometimes main stalk of bunch diseased. The bunch becomes black and rotten.
- Acervuli produces cylindrical conidiophores, hyaline, septate, branched.
- Conidia hyaline, non-septate, oval to elliptical.

5. Bunchy top : *Banana bunchy top virus*

Diagnostic Symptoms

- Plants are extremely stunted .
- Dark broken bands of green tissues on the veins, leaves and petioles.
- Leaves are reduced in size marginal chlorosis and curling.
- Leaves upright and become brittle.
- Many leaves are crowded at the top.
- Branches size will very small. If infected earlier no bunch will be produced.

Crop stage wise IDM activities in Banana		
Crop stage	Diseases	Step wise IDM practices
Pre planting/Planting	Soil borne pathogens, nematodes	• Deep ploughing during summer. • Use of disease free planting material. • Storage of large corms in the sun for two weeks prior to planting. • Select healthy suckers. • Avoid growing Robusta, Karpooruvally, Malbhog, Champa and Adukkar. • Grow less susceptible varieties like Poovan, Kadali, Kunnan, Poomkalli. • Intercropping of banana with *Crotalaria juncea*, marigold reduces burrowing nem. • Crop rotation with non-host crops.
Vegetative stage	Sigatoka	• Removal and destruction of the affected leaves. • Prevent water accumulation around the plant and go for periodical weeding. • Select tolerant varieties such as Ney Poovan, Pachanadan, Karpuravalli, Fhia 1 (Gold fi nger), Sannachenkadali. • Chemical control: Spray Propiconazole 25% EC @ 0.1% (100 ml/100 l water.) in 200-400 l of water/ acre. or Copper oxychloride 50% WP @ 1Kg in 300-400 l of water/acre.
	Moko	• Providing good drainage. • Disinfestation of tools with formaldehyde diluted with water in 1:3 ratio. • Crop rotation (3 years rotation with sugarcane or rice) & providing good drainage. • Allow fallow period or flooding during off -season.
	Bunchy top	• Select suckers from disease free areas. • Infected plants are destroyed using 4ml of 2, 4, D (50g in 400 ml of water). • Remove weeds which are attractant to aphids. • Select tolerant varieties such as Poovan, Pachanadan. • Aphids are controlled by using sprays of insecticidal like Imidacloprid 0.05% or other approved pesticides. Soapy water and oil sprays can kill aphids on contact. Aphid control should be a regular, long-term practice. Do not chop diseased plants with aphids because the aphids will fly away to infect other plants. .

	Panama	• Avoid growing of susceptible cultivars *viz.*, Rasthali, Monthan, Red banana and Virupakshi. • Grow resistant cultivar Poovan. • Removal and destruction of aff ected leaves followed by spraying with BM (1%) +linseed oil (2%). • Select tolerant varieties such as Dwarf Cavendish, Robusta, Fhia 1 (Gold fi nger), Anai komban, Nivedya Kadali.
	Anthracnose	• Proper sanitation of handling and prompt cooling to 14° C are essential in minimising the disease in cold storage..
	Tip rot	• Remove infected plants and destroy. • Drench with Carbendazim + Mancozeb 75% WP @ 600-800 g in 400 l of water/acre.
	Infectious chlorosis	• Destroy infected plants. • Use disease free suckers. • Dry heat treatment of suckers at 40° C for 1 day. • Avoid growing cucurbits as intercrop. • Aphids are controlled by using sprays of insecticidal like Imidacloprid 0.05% or other approved pesticides. Soapy water and oil sprays can kill aphids on contact. Aphid control should be a regular, long-term practice. Do not chop diseased plants with aphids because the aphids will fly away to infect other plants.
	Banana bract mosaic virus/ streak mosaic	• Dry heat treatment of suckers at 40° C for 1 day. • Avoid growing cucurbits as intercrop.
Reproductive stage (5th-7th month):	Anthracnose	• Proper sanitation of handling and prompt cooling to 14° C are essential in minimising the disease in cold storage.

19.13 IDM in Grapes

Sl.No	Name of Disease	Causal organism
1	Downy mildew	*Plasmopara viticola*
2	Powdery mildew	*Uncinula necator*
3	Bird's Eye Spot/Anthracnose	*Gloeosporium ampelophagum* (*Elsinoe ampelina)*

Major diseases and their diagnostic symptoms

1. Downy Mildew: *Plasmopara viticola*

Diagnostic Symptoms

- Symptoms appear on all aerial and tender parts of the vine.
- Irregular, yellowish, translucent spots on the upper surface of the leaves.
- Correspondingly on the lower surface, dirty white, powdery growth of fungus appears.
- Affected leaves become, yellow and brown and gets dried due to necrosis.
- Premature defoliation.
- Dwarfing of tender shoots.
- Infected leaves, shoots and tendrils are covered by whitish growth of the fungus.
- White growth of fungus on berries which subsequently becomes leathery and shrivels. Infected berries turn hard, bluish green and then brown.
- Later infection of berries results in soft rot symptoms. Normally, the fully grown or maturing berries do not contact fresh infection as stomata turn non-functional.
- No cracking of the skin of the berries.

2. Powdery Mildew : *Uncinula necator*

Diagnostic Symptoms

- Powdery growth mostly on the upper surface of the leaves.
- Malformation and discolouration of affected leaves.
- Discolouration of stem to dark brown.
- Floral infection results in shedding of flowers and poor fruit set.
- Early berry infection results in shedding of affected berries.
- Powdery growth is visible on older berries and the infection results in the cracking of skin of the berries.

3. Anthracnose/Bird's Eye Spot: *Gloeosporium ampelophagum* (*Elsinoe ampelina)*

Diagnostic Symptoms

- Symptoms visible on leaves, stem, tendrils and berries.
- Young shoots and fruits are more susceptible than leaves.
- Circular, greyish black spots or red spots with yellow halo appear.
- Later the centre of the spot becomes grey, sunken and fall off resulting in a symptom called 'shot hole'.
- Black, sunken lesions appear on young shoots.
- Cankerous lesions on older shoots. Girdling and death of shoots occur.
- Infection on the stalk of bunches and berries result in the shedding of bunches and berries respectively.
- Sunken spots with ashy grey centre and dark margin on fruits (Birds eye symptom).
- Mummification and shedding of berries.

Crop stage wise IDM activities in Grape		
Crop stage	**Diseases**	**Step wise IDM practices**
Pre planting stage	Soil borne pathogens, nematodes	• Deep ploughing of fields during summer to control nematodes population and popagules of soil borne pathogens. • Soil solarization can be done for sterilizing the nursery mixture. • Timely sowing should be done. • Field sanitation, rogueing. • Destroy the alternate host plants as well as crop debris. • Crop rotation with non-cereals. • Adopt ecological engineering by growing the attractant, repellent, and trap crops around the field bunds.

Planting stage	Root-knot nematode	• Intercropping of marigold reduces nematode population. • Nursery should be raised in nematode free sites or fumigated or solarized beds. • Repellant plants: Marigold. • Follow common cultural practices. • Application of decomposed poultry manure @ 200g / sq. m.
	Leaf blight/ Anthracnose	• Irrigation by rose can. • Avoid water stress and water stagnation conditions. • Use of resistant varieties such as– Bangalore Blue, Beauty Seedless,Bharat Early, Golden queen, Large white. • Spray Aureofungin 46.15%w/v. SP@ 0.005%, 300 l/acre or chlorothalonil 75% WP@ 0.2% or 200 g in 100lof water /acre or iprodione 50% WP@ 0.4-0.8 Kg in 200 l of water/acre or kitazin 48% EC @ 0.20%or 200 ml in 200 l of water.
Vegetative stage	Powdery mildew	• Cultural practices that reduce humidity within the vineyard, enable good air circulation through the canopy, and provide good light exposure to all leaves and clusters aid in managing powdery mildew. • Use an under vine irrigation system and manage it carefully, excess can favour the disease. • Chemical control: Spray hexaconazole 2 % SC @ 0.6-1.2 l in 200-300 l of water/acre or hexaconazole 5% EC@ 200-400 ml in 200 l of water/acre or kresoxim-methyl 44.3% SC@ 240-280 ml in 200 l of water/acre or lime sulphur 22% SC @ 0.8-1 l/acre or myclobutanil 10% WP @ 0.04%, 200 l /acre or penconazole 10% EC@ 50ml/100Lt. water or triadimefon 25% WP@ 0.010% in 300 l of water, depending upon the requirement.
	Downy mildew	• Pruning of the vines after the second week of october helps to minimize the damage by this disease. • All affected portions of the vine should be removed at the time of pruning and destroyed immediately. • Downy mildew infected leaves should be selectively collected and disposed in compost pit.

		• Chemical control:Aureofungin46.15%w/v. SP@ 0.005% or chlorothalonil 75% WP@ 0.2% or copper oxychloride 50% WG@ 0.24% or cymoxanil50%WP@ 0.25% depending upon the crop stage and equipment used or cyazafamid 34.5% SC@ 80 ml in 200 l of water/acre or dimethomorph50%WP @ 400 g in 300 l of water/acre or fosetyl-AL 80% WP @ 560-800 g in 300- 400 l of water/ acre or kresoxim-methyl 44.3% SC@ 240-280 ml in 200 l of water/acre or cymoxanil 8%+ Mancozeb 64%WP @ 600-800 g in 200-400 l of water/acre or famoxadone 16.6%+ Cymoxanil22.1%SC @ 200 ml in 200-300 l of water/acre or fenamidone4.44%+ Fosetyl AI 66.7%WG@ 800-1000 g in 200-300l of water/acre or fenamidone10%+ mancozeb 50%WDG @ 600 g in 200-300 l of water/ acre or metalaxyl M 4%+ mancozeb 64% WP @ 200-400 l/acre of 0.25% or metalaxyl8%+ mancozeb 64% WP@ 200 l/acre of 0.5% or metiram 55% + pyraclostrobin 5% WG @ 600-700 g in 300 l of water/acre.
	Anthracnose, Blight	• Prophylactic measures should be followed for effective control. • All affected twigs or canes showing cankers should be removed while pruning. • The pruned twigs and leaves should be burnt or buried deep in the soil. • Chemical control: Same as sowing stage.
	Bitter rot and Bacterial leaf spot, Rust	• Collecting and burning the infected plant parts minimizes the spread of the disease. • Increase air circulation in the vineyard. • Remove disease cane from the vineyard during normal pruning operations in the dormant season. • Follow up hand pruning.

Flowering & Fruiting stage	Powdery mildew, Downy mildew	• Remove abnormal un-harvested bunches from vines and burn them. • Remove all shoots emerging from the crown near ground. • Shoots hanging from trellises towards ground should be tied on trellises or can be removed if they are extra. • Chemical control: Same as vegetative stage
	Blight, Anthracnose, Bitter rot and Bacterial leaf spot	• Promote good air circulation and light penetration by controlling weeds and suckers, proper pruning, and positioning or removing shoots for uniform leaf development. • Where possible, rows should be planted in the direction of the prevailing wind. Good air circulation and light penetration will promote faster drying of plant parts and reduce disease incidence. • Prevent wounding of berries by controlling insects, birds and other grape diseases.
	Botrytis rot	• Careful handling in the field, pre-cooling and refrigeration helps in controlling the disease. • Pruning and thinning of the vineyard reduces humidity around the clusters..
	Blue rot	• Avoiding injuries to the ripe berries helps to reduce soft rot. • Clean planting stock; (i) Disease wood removal and immediate burning;• (ii) fungicide application at shoot extension and later if temperatures are cool.
Postharvest	Black mould rot, Blue mould rot, Green mould rot, Botrytis rot	• Careful handling and prompt refrigeration to 1-2 ºC or below prevents the disease in storage. • Inclusion of sulphur di oxide releasing pads in the boxes while packing helps to control the disease.
	Rhizopus rot	• Inclusion of sulphur di oxide releasing pads in the boxes 2 while packing, removing of diseased berries during grading, avoiding injury to the berries while packing and handling helps to restrict the growth of fungi. • Avoiding injuries to the ripe berries helps to reduce soft rot. • Maintaining cold storage temperature. between 40-10 ºC prevents fungal growth.

19.14 IDM in Citrus

Sl.No	Name of Disease	Causal organism
1	Gummosis	*Phytophthora parasitica, P. palmivora, P. citrophthora*
2	Canker	*Xanthomonas campestris pv citri*
3	Scab/Verucosis	*Elsinoe fawcett*
4	Tristeza or Quick decline	*Citrus tristeza virus*
5	Greening	*Liberobactor asiaticum*
6	Exocortis of scaly butt	Viroid

Major diseases and their diagnostic symptoms

1. Gummosis : *Phytophthora parasitica, P. palmivora, P. citrophthora*

Diagnostic Symptoms

- First symptoms are dark staining of bark which progresses into the wood.
- Bark at the base is destroyed resulting in girdling and finally death of the tree.
- Bark in such parts dries, shrinks and cracks and shreds in lengthwise vertical strips.
- Later profuse exudation of gum from the bark of the trunk(characteristic symptom).
- The infection spreads both upward to the leaves and even fruits and downward to the roots causing fibrous root rot.
- The fibrous root rot destroys a major portion of the root system.
- However, the trunck and root infections may usually result in ultimate drying of the tree.

2. Canker : *Xanthomonas campestris* pv *citri*

Diagnostic Symptoms

- The disease appears as raised , rough, corky brownish pustules with characteristic halo on leaves.
- Canker lesions on the fruit do not possess the yellow halo as on leaves.
- Several lesions on fruit may coalesce to form a patch. The crater-like appearance is more marked on fruits than on leaves.
- On fruits, canker lesions reduce market value.
- The plants are also stunted and fruit yields are reduced considerably.

3. Scab/Verucosis : *Elsinoe fawcett*

Diagnostic Symptoms

- The disease is first noticed by the irregular, corky spots on the leaves, twigs and fruits.

- The spot may be a few mm up to one cm in diameter.
- They become warty, erupted with cracks and scabby, hence the name.
- On the fruits the warty growth are surrounded by yellowish or chlorotic haloes.
- The color of the spot turns from yellow to orange –brown and finally black.
- Several spots run together to form large patches of corky outgrowths.
- The scab may be a few or many on each fruits and the market value of the fruits is considerably reduced because of the infection

4. Tristeza or Quick Decline : *Citrus tristeza virus* (CTV)

Diagnostic Symptoms

- The infected trees usually show general decline.
- Leaves becomes dull and chlorotic and twigs start drying from tip downwards.
- In sweet orange or mandarin on susceptible root stocks, leaves develop deficiency symptoms and abscise.
- Roots decay, twigs die back. Fruit set diminishes; only skeleton remains.
- Fine pitting of inner face of bark of sour orange stock.
- Acid lime leaves show large number of vein flecks (elongated translucent area).
- Tree stunted and dies yield very much reduced. Fruits are small in size.

5. **Greening or Huanglongbin**: *Liberibacter asiaticus (Phloem limited Bacterium)*

Diagnostic Symptoms

- The disease initiates as interveinal chlorosis and leads to the complete yellowing of the leaf with few green islands.
- Secondary growth is upright, short with small leaves and multiple buds.
- Leaf symptom pattern indicates zinc or iron deficiency.
- The fruits also show conspicuous sun blotching with yellow discoloration.
- As the disease advances, the plant shows severe die back symptoms.

6. Exocortis of scaly butt : *Viroid*

Diagnostic Symptoms

- Vertical cracking and scaling of bark in the entire, root stock.
- Extreme stunting of plant.
- Affects only rangpur lime, trifoliate orange and citrange root stocks.

Crop stage wise IDM activities in Citrus		
Crop stage	Diseases	Step wise IDM practices
Pre planting/ Planting	Soil borne pathogens, nematodes	• Deep summer ploughing of field reduces the incidence of soil-borne pathogens. • Pits of 1 meter cube are dug in square system during. summer season and kept open for controlling soil borne diseases. • Rogue out diseased seedling. • Use resistant/tolerant varieties. • Destroy the alternate host plants.
Vegetative growth and fruiting stage	Scab	• Collect and destroy the infested leaves, twigs and fruits. • Spray with 0.3 % COC or 1.0% Bordeaux mixture or 0.2% chlorothalonil at 15 day interval.
	Canker	• Select seedlings free from canker for planting in main field. • Prune out and burn all canker infected twigs before monsoon. • Maintain proper aeration by training and pruning for reducing the leaf wetness period. • Spray Streptomycin Sulphate 9% + Tetracycline Hydrocloride 1%) or Spray Streptocycline 50 to100 ppm solution repeatedly at an interval of 15 to20 days after the appearance of new growth. • Cover the foliage and young fruits fully.
	Citrus Tristeza	• Use certified budwood free of CTV. • Remove all diseased trees as and when the disease is noticed. • Fresh plantings to be taken with virus free materials on tolerant rootstocks. • For sweet orange and mandarin avoid susceptible rootstocks. • For acid lime, use seedling immunised with mild strain of Citrus tristeza virus (Cross protection). • Periodic sprays of insecticides like Imidacloprid 0.05 % controls the population of citrus aphids that reduces secondary spread of the disease in the orchard. • Spray Copper oxy chloride 50% WP @ 1 kg in 300-400 l of water/acre.

	Gummosis	• Remove diseased bark and a buffer strip of healthy, light brown to greenish bark around the margins of the infection. • Preventive measures like selection of proper site with adequate drainage. • Use of resistant rootstocks and avoiding contact of water with the tree trunk by adopting ring method of irrigation are effective. • Spray Aureofungin 46.15% w/v. SP @ 300 (1%) gm / ml/acre.
	Greasy spot	• Spray Zineb 75% WP @ 0.25% , if required repeat after 15 days.
	Greening	• Use resistant sour orange rootstocks for propagating economic varieties. • Use certified pathogen free bud wood for propagation. • Selection of proper site with adequate drainage and high budding (30 to 46 cm or above). • Provision of an inner ring about 45 cm around the tree trunk to prevent moist soil. (Double ring method of irrigation). • Avoid irrigation water from coming in direct contact with the tree trunk. • Avoid injuries to crown roots or base of stem during cultural operations. • Control psyllids with insecticides like imidacloprid . • Applying Bordeaux paste or ZnSO4, CuSO4, lime (5:1:4) to a height of about 60 cm above the ground level at least once a year.
	Brown rot	• Spray Captan 75% WP@500 g in 6-8 l of water/acre.

19.15 IDM in Guava

Sl. No	Disease	Pathogen
1	Wilt	*Fusaium oxysporum* f sp *psidii, F. solani*
2	Anthracnose	*Colletotrichum gloeosporioides* (*Glomerella psidii)*
3	Canker	*Pestalotia psidii*

Major diseases and their diagnostic symptoms

1. Wilt – *Fusaium oxysporum* f.sp. *psidii*

Diagnostic Symptoms

- The symptoms are browning and wilting of leaves, discoloration of the stem and death of the branches along one side.
- Sometimes the infection girdles the entire stem and the whole plant wilts.

- The laves fall off and plant may die in the course of a year or more.
- When an infected stem is cut open the tissues extending up to the cambium region display a dark color.
- The fungus is present in the stem tissues, especially at the basal portions near the ground level.

2. Anthracnose: *Colletotrichum gloeosporioides* (*Glomerella psidii)*

Diagnostic Symptoms

- Symptoms of this disease are observed on mature fruits on the tree.
- The characteristic symptoms consist of sunken, dark colored, necrotic lesions. Under humid conditions, the necrotic lesions become covered with pinkish spore masses.
- As the disease progresses, the small sunken lesions coalesce to form large necrotic patches affecting the flesh of the fruit.
- The infected area in the unripe fruits become corky and often develops cracks in case of severe infection.
- On ripe fruit, the infection causes softening of tissue and lesions attains a diameter of 10 to 20 mm infection.

3. Canker: *Pestalotia psidii*

Diagnostic Symptoms

- The disease generally occurs on green fruits and rarely on leaves.
- Appearance of minute, brown or rust colored, circular, necrotic areas on fruits which in advanced stage of infection tears open the epidermis in a circinate manner.
- The margin of lesion is elevated and as depressed area is noticeable inside.
- The crater like appearance is noticeable on fruits than on leaves.
- The canker is confined to a very shallow area and does not penetrates deep into the flesh of the fruit.
- In older cankers, fruiting bodies of white mycelium consisting of numerous spores are noticeable.
- The infected fruit remain underdeveloped, become hard, malformed and mummified and great in numbers.

Crop stage wise IDM activities in Guava		
Crop stage	Diseases	Step wise IDM practices
Pre planting / Planting stage	Soil borne pathogens and nematodes	• Deep ploughing of fields during summer to control nematodes population, to expose popagules of soil borne pathogens. • Soil solarization can be done for sterilizing the nursery mixture. • Timely sowing should be done. • Field sanitation, rogueing. • Destroy the alternate host plants as well as crop debris. • Crop rotation with non-cereals. • Ploughing the field before digging the pits.
Vegetative stage		• Destroy crop debris. • Avoid water logging. • Avoid water stress. • Green manuring during rainy season. • Grow leguminous crops or vegetables as intercrops during the first three years of planting, provided irrigation facility is available. • Fertilizers should be applied based on soil test values and recommendation for the agro-ecological regions.
Flowering & Fruiting stage	Wilt	• Follow clean cultivation and strict sanitation in orchard. • Wilted trees should be uprooted, burnt and trench should be dug around the tree trunk. • Roots of plants should not be damaged while transplanting.
Flowering & Fruiting stage		• Maintain proper tree vigour by timely and adequately manuring inter-culture and irrigation enable them to withstand infection. • The pits may be treated with formalin and kept covered for about 3 days and transplanting should be done after two weeks. • Apply organic manures, oil cakes and lime. • Use rootstocks resistant to wilt i.e. Cross of Psidium molle x *P. guajava*. • Eco-friendly approach of guava wilt control is suggested where biological control (Trichoderma spp., *Aspergillus niger* AN27), soil amendment (lime, neem cakes, gypsum) and intercropping (marigold, turmeric) are effective.
	Fruit rot/ fruit canker/ algal leaf and fruit spot	• Prune and destroy the dead twigs and fruits. • Plant spacing and fertilizer régimes should be managed to avoid unnecessarily dense plant canopy. • Prune old and non-productive branch which may serve as potential source of infection.

		• For managing fruit rot disease good field sanitation (maintain field free of infected dry or semi-dry twigs and mummified fruits of previous harvest which may serve as primary inoculum. • Algal leaf spot can be reduced by maintaining tree vigour with cultural techniques such as proper fertilization and irrigation, proper pruning to enhance air circulation within the canopy and sunlight penetration, managing weeds and wider tree spacing. • Chemical control: Apply Zineb 75% WP @600 -800 g in 300-400 l of water/ acre or Mancozeb 75% WP+ Carbendazim 50% WP @ 20g in 10 l of water/tree.
	Dieback/ Anthracnose/ Stem canker and dry fruit rot	• Maintain orchard hygienic. • Monitor disease and use of micro irrigation systems. • Follow clean cultivation and strict sanitation in orchard. • Use disease free planting material. • Implement a good weed control to reduce humidity. • Adhere to recommended plant density to reduce competition for sunlight, water and nutrient.
Post-harvest	Diseases	• Keeping of good quality of fruits and bagging fruits. • Remove and destroy all the affected fruits to reduce, the incidence of Anar butterfly. • Cover the fruit with polythene bags when the fruits are up to 5 cm.

19.16 IDM in Papaya

Sl.No	Name of disease	Causal Organism
1	Stem rot / Foot rot	*Pythium aphanidermatum*
2	Powdery mildew	*Oidium caricae*
3	Anthracnose	*Colletotrichum gleoesporiodes*
4	Ring spot	*Papaya ring spot virus*
5	Leaf curl	*Nicotiana virus 10*

Major diseases and their diagnostic symptoms

1. Stem rot / Foot rot/Collar rot – *Pythium aphanidermatum*

Diagnostic Symptoms

- Spongy ,water soaked spot in the stem at the ground level which enlarge and griddle the stem.
- The diseased area turns brown or black and rot.
- Rotting generally spreads above and below on the stem down to the roots which also begin to rot.
- Terminal leaves turn yellow droop off.
- The entire plant topples over and dies.
- Common in 2-3 year old plants.

2. Powdery Mildew – *Oidium caricae*

Diagnostic Symptoms

- White powdery growth on the under surface of the infected leaves.
- Leaves show blotches of yellow or pale green look near the veins at the infection spots which are surrounded by normal green colored tissues.
- Under severe attacks, the top portion of the seedlings may die and the fruit yield is reduced.

3. Anthracnose – *Colletotrichum gloeosporioides*

Diagnostic Symptoms

- Spots on fruits appear as brown superficial discolouration of the skin.
- Spots develop into circular, slightly sunken areas and 1 to 3 cm in diameter.
- Lesions coalesce and sparse mycelial growth appears on the margins of the spots.
- Early fruit infection results in mummification and deformation.
- Necrotic spots on leaves and stems.
- Older parts are generally highly susceptible.

4. Papaya Ring Spot – *Papaya ring spot virus*

Diagnostic Symptoms

- Vein clearing, puckering and chlorophyll leaf tissues lobbing in.
- Margin and distal parts of leaves roll downward and inwards, mosaic mottling, dark green blisters, leaf distortion which result in shoe string system and stunting of plants.
- On fruits circular concentric rings are produced. If affected earlier no fruit formation.
- Vectored by aphids *Aphis gossypii, A. craccivora* and also spreads to cucurbits not through seeds.

5. Leaf curl – *Papaya leaf curl virus*

Diagnostic Symptoms

- Curling, crinkling and distortion of leaves, reduction of leaf lamina, rolling of leaf margins inward and downward, thickening of veins.
- Leaves become leathery, brittle and distorted. Plants stunted. Affected plants does not produce flowers and fruits.
- Spread by whitefly *Bemisia tabaci.*

Crop stage wise IDM activities in Papaya		
Crop stage	Diseases	Step wise IDM practices
Pre planting / Planting stage	Soil borne pathogens and nematodes	• Deep ploughing of fields during summer. • Soil solarization. • Timely sowing should be done. • Field sanitation, rogueing. • Destroy the alternate host plants. • Apply manures and fertilizers as per soil test. recommendations. • Crop rotation with graminaceous crops. • Intercropping of marigold reduces nematode population. • Nursery should be raised in nematode free sites or fumigated or solarized beds. • Apply neem cake @ 100 Kg/acre at the time of transplanting for reducing nematodes .
Sowing/ Seedling	Soil borne diseases, Nematodes	• Seedling raised in insect proof conditions. • Two month old seedling is ready for transplanting. • Papaya don't withstand water logging, hence well drained upland fields should be selected for cultivation. • Under drip, ring method should be followed. • Remove and destroy virus infected seedlings/plants. • Apply neem seed kernel extract (NSKE) 5%/groundnut oil @ 1-2% on to the plants to manage the vector population.

		• Use resistant/tolerant varieties. • Sowing should be completed within recommended periods. • Intercropping with sunnhemp or marigold or daincha.
Vegetative/ Flowering/ Maturity stage	Foot Rot	• The crop should be irrigated by adopting the ring method of irrigation so that the water does not come in direct contact with the stem. • Avoid water logging.
	Anthracnose	• Diseased leaves, twigs, gall midge infected leaves and fruits, should be collected and burnt. • Covering the fruits on trees, 15 days prior to harvest with news or brown paper bags.
	Powdery mildews	• Prune diseased leaves to reduce primary inoculum load. • Keep proper spacing during sowing. • Spray (Thiophanate methyl 70% WP @ 0.1% along with sticker @ 0.05%)
	Papaya mosaic virus	• Good field sanitation such as removal and destruction of affected plant reduce the spread of the disease.
	Papaya leaf curl virus	• Uproot the virus affected plants • Avoid growing tomato, tobacco near papaya. • Control whitefly vector. • Removal and destruction of the affected plants is the only control measure to reduce the spread of the disease.
	Papaya ring spot virus	• Use of yellow sticky strap to control of aphid vector. • Use of resistant varieties. • Early detection of infected plants and prompt removal can check the spread of the disease. • Rogue out infected plants of papaya as early as possible to avoid further infection within the field.
Post-harvest	Anthracnose, Stem end rot, Aspergillus rot, Rhizopus rot, Fruit rot, Phomopsis	• Avoid harvesting of immature fruits. • Cool fruits immediately after harvest and store in well ventilated containers. • The disease can be checked by sorting the fruit at 100 °C or below but the rot appears after 2-3 days when such fruits are brought back to 20°C or above. • Hot water treatment at 49 °C for 20 min. • Postharvest dip treatment of fruits with botanical fungicides could also control the diseases during storage.

19.17 IDM in Apple

Sl.No	Name of diseases	Causal organism
1	Apple scab	*Venturia inaequalis* (Cooke) Wint
2	Black rot and canker	*Botryosphaeria obtuse* Schw
3	Collar rot	*Phytophthora cactorum* Lebert & Cohn
4	Powdery mildew	*Podosphaera leucotricha* Ellis & Everh
5	Sooty blotch and fly speck:	*Schizothyrium pomi* (Mont. & Fr.) Arx
6	Apple mosaic and other virus diseases	Apple mosaic virus, Apple chlorotic leaf spot virus

Major diseases and their diagnostic symptoms

1. Apple Scab

- Scab may appear on leaves, fruits, petioles and green twigs.
- The most striking symptoms of scab are commonly observed on leaves and fruits.
- Fruits may show small, rough, black, circular lesions on their skin while on the tree or after keeping in cold storage.
- Fruits picked from the infected trees are too sticky to keep even in cold storage they appear apparently healthy.
- Such fruits soon develop scab symptoms even at low temperature and may not last long in storage.
- The affected fruits rot due to secondary infection of the lesions.
- Secondary infections on leaves are so numerous that the entire surface of the leaf appears covered with scab, commonly referred to as sheet scab.
- Lesions on young fruits resemble those on leaves but turn dark brown to black and become corky or scab like with time.
- Infections are often limited to one or two spots per fruit, secondary infections are clumped together.

2. Powdery Mildew

- The disease infects leaves, blossoms, green shoots and the fruit.
- On leaves, the fungus appears as felt like patches or as a solid mat on the surface, particularly on their undersurfaces.
- Initial infections on the underside of the leaf may cause chlorotic patches or spots to occur on the upper surface.
- Infected leaves tend to crinkle, curl or roll upwards along the edges, giving them a narrow appearance.
- During severe infection, leaves will usually drop prematurely during the summer.

- Infected shoots are stunted.
- Severe infection leads to defoliation of the mildewed shoots with a subsequent curtailment of its growth and reduction in number of its potential buds.
- Small greyish or white patches are seen on the underside of leaves. Diseased twigs are crinkled. Fruits show stunted growth along with typical rosetting.

3. Blotch

- Disease appears both on leaves and fruits.
- Dark brown patches develop on upper surface of leaves varying from 5-10 cm dia. as typical blotch symptoms.
- Under favourable climatic conditions, these spots coalesce to form large dark brown blotches and the surrounding areas turn yellow.
- This yellowing advances towards petiole and induces mid-season defoliation.
- Irregular necrotic blotches on mature leaves characterize the disease.
- In affected orchards, apple fruits nearing maturity are commonly seen hanging on the defoliated trees.
- Repeated pre-mature leaf shedding results in failure of the crop in the following season.
- Golden delicious varieties are most severely affected.

4. Canker Disease Complex

- With the increase in the area under apple cultivation, a number of new canker diseases have appeared.
- Stem and branch cankers cause huge losses through girdling of branches, limbs and die-back of twigs resulting in death of plants.
- Six types of cankers viz, silver leaf canker, smoky blight canker, pink canker, stem canker, nail head canker and stem black canker are important in India.

5. White Root Rot

- This is a soil borne-disease causing death of the plants and is an increasingly important problem.
- Lateral roots turn dark brown and become infected with white flocculent fungus during monsoon months.
- Bronzing of leaves, stunted growth and size are important above-ground symptoms.
- Root rot affected trees are usually associated with a heavy blossom and fruiting next year, however, in succeeding years, few leaves emerge and much of the immature fruits fail to reach maturity.
- Infected trees often persist for 2-3 years depending upon infestation of fungus.

6. Replant Disease Complex

- It is a complex malady characterized by suppressed growth of young trees in old orchard sites.
- It is referred to as soil sickness due to many biotic factors and soil starvation due to abiotic factors.
- It has no symptoms other than stunted growth of trees during the first few years of planting.
- Affected trees leaf out each spring vigorously with no shoot growth with fewer leaves, which are often smaller than healthy plant.

7. Collar Rot

- This disease is also known as crown rot causing extensive losses.
- The above ground symptoms are often confused with white root rot.
- The infection starts from the collar region and spreads to the underground parts. Bark at the soil level becomes slimy and rots resulting in cankered areas.
- The attacked trees are recognized by chlorotic foliage with red colouration of veins and margins.

Crop stage wise IDM activities in Apple		
Crop stage	Diseases	Step wise IDM practices
Pre planting/ Planting	Soil borne pathogens, nematodes and resting stages of pathogens	• Pits of 1 meter cube are dug in square system during summer season and kept open for controlling soil born pests. • Soils of different horizons should be analysed to know the inherent fertility and soil condition of the fi eld. • The fertilizer dose should be based upon soil fertility, type of soil, kind and age of trees, cultural practices, climate and crop load. • Application of manures and fertilizers start right from planting of an orchard at the time of filling of pits. • In an orchard of optimal fertility, N, P and K may be applied in the ratio 70: 30: 70 g/year/ tree.

	Soil borne pathogens and other diseases	• Grow resistant/tolerant varieties *viz.*, Emra, Red Free, Ambstraking, Ambroyal, Ambrich and Ambred in the endemic areas for controlling scab and Maharaji Chunth and Golden Chinese (apple cultivars),Yantarka Altaskya, Dolgoe (crab apple cultivars) for controlling powdery mildew disease
	Scab and powdery mildew	• Use healthy infestation-free plants. • Aphids usually spread through infested stocks, avoid planting infested stocks.
Vegetative stage	White rot/root rot	• For root rot, make 5-10 trunk injections fungicide @ 2 g/tree.
Reproductive		
Tight cluster stage	Scab	• Clean cultivation, collection and destruction of fallen leaves and pruned materials in winter to prevent the sexual cycle. • Collect and burn the infected plant debris. • Follow proper trimming and pruning of twigs and branches followed by burning. • Apply urea (2 Kg/acre at pre-leaf fall stage spring and dolomitic lime (2.5 ton/acre) in autumn over fallen leaves to accelerate decomposition. • Chemical control: Spray bitertanol 25% WP @ 0.75 g/l of water and use spray fl uid of 10 l/tree or chlorothalonil 75% WP@ 200 g in 100 l of water and 10 l of spray fluid/tree or difenaconazole 25 EC @ 15 ml in 100 l of water or dodine 65% WP @ 0.75 g/l and use spray fluid of 10 l of spray fluid/tree or fenarimol 12% EC @ 40 ml in 100 l of water and 10 l of spray fl uid/tree or flusilazole 40% EC @ 0.1 ml/l of water and 10 l of spray fluid/acre or hexaconazole 5% EC @ 50 ml/100 l of water or myclobutanil 10% WP @ 0.4 ml/l of water and use spray fluid of 10 l/tree or penconazole 10% EC @ 50 ml in 100 l of water and 10 l of spray fluid/tree or thiophanate methyl 70% WP @ 286 g in 300-400 l of water/acre.
Pink bud stage	Scab and core rot	• Same as above.
	Powdery mildew	• Sanitation of orchard. • Use resistant varieties. • Removal of over wintering infected terminals by pruning (6-8" below the infection) is good for reducing the inoculum. • Practice trimming and pruning to reduce the humidity.

		• Spray aureofungin 46.15% w/v SP @ 0.5 ml/l of water and use spray fluid of 10 l/tree or lime sulphur 22% SC @ 800-2000 ml/acre (use 2% pre-blossom and 1% postblossom or sulphur 80% WP @ 1000-2000 g in 300- 400 l of water/ acre.
Petal fall/pea stage	Scab, Powdery mildew and Alternaria blight	• Same as above.
Fruit development (Walnut size)	Scab, Marssonina blotch and Alternaria blight	• Same as above.
Pre-harvest stage (20-25 days before harvest)	Scab, Marssonina blotch, Alternaria blight, Sooty blotch and fly speck, Bitter rot and brown rot	• Cultural practices same as above. • For sooty blotch, spray Mancozeb 75% WG + Carbendazim 50 %@ 3 g/l of water and use spray fl uid of 10 l/tree. • For fly speck, spray captan 75% WP @ 666.8 g/ acre in water required to distribute 10-20 l/tree • For bitter rot, spray or difenoconazole 25 EC @ 15 ml in 100 l of water (spray volume depending upon the tree size and spray equipment used)
Post-harvest	Scab, other diseases	• Same as above.
	Bitter rot, Brown rot	• Same as above.
Dormant stage	Scab and other foliar diseases	• Same as above.
	Black rot/Canker	• Proper pruning should be done to avoid mechanical injury. • Use *Trichoderma viride* or *T. harzianum* with neem cake.
	White rot/Root rot	• For root rot, make 5-10 trunk injections @ 2 g/ tree.

19.18 IDM in Coconut

Sl. No	Disease	Causal Organism
1	Bud rot	*Phytophthora palmivora*
2	Stem bleeding	*Ceratocystis paradoxa/ Ophiostoma paradoxa*
3	Grey blight	*Pestalotiopsis palmarum*
4	Basal stem rot (Thanjavur wilt / Bole rot)	*Ganoderma lucidum*

Major diseases and their diagnostic symptoms

1. Bud Rot - *Phytophthora palmivora*

Diagnostic Symptoms

- Severe on young palms.
- Yellowish green discoloration of the heart leaf or crown leaf.
- The basal tissues of the leaf rot quickly and can be easily separated from the crown.
- Spindle withers and droop down.
- Older leaves develop irregular, water soaked spots which are sunken in nature.
- The leaves and sheath in the central spindle fall off leaving an outer whorl of green leaves.
- The withered central shoot can be pulled out very easily from the crown.
- The central crown may rot and in few months the tree may wilt.
- Young nuts fail to mature and fall.

2. Stem bleeding – *Ceratocystis paradoxa/ Ophiostoma paradoxa*

Diagnostic Symptoms

- The characteristic symptom is the exudation of reddish brown fluid from the cracks in the stem.
- The fluid trickles down to several feet on the stem and the exudates dries up forming a black crust. The tissues below the cracks turn yellow and decay. As the disease progresses, more area underneath the bark gets decayed and the bleeding patch extends further up.
- The vigour of the tree is affected and nut yield is reduced.
- The tree is not killed out right but become uneconomical to maintain.
- In extreme cases, the trees may become barren and die.

3. Grey Blight – *Pestalotiopsis palmarum*

Diagnostic Symptoms

- Disease symptoms develop in mature leaves of outer whorl.

- Minute yellow spots surrounded by a grayish margin appear on leaflets. Gradually, the centre of the spots turns grayish white with dark brown margins and a yellow halo.
- Spots coalesce into irregular necrotic patches.
- Complete drying and shrivelling of leaf blade occur giving a blighted or burnt appearance.
- Large number of globose or ovoid black acervuli appears on the upper surface of affected leaves.

4. Basal Stem Rot (Thanjavur wilt / Bole rot) ; *Ganoderma lucidum*

Diagnostic Symptoms

- The most usual symptoms are yellowing, withering and drooping of the outer fronds which remain hanging around the trunk for several months before shedding.
- The younger leaves remain green for sometime and later turn yellowish brown.
- The new fronds produced become successively smaller and yellowish in colour which do not unfold properly.
- The wilting plants also show bleeding patches near the base of the trunk.
- A brown gummy liquid oozes out from the cracks in the tree which slowly result in the death of outer tissues.
- As the infection advances, fresh bleeding patches appear above the old once, up to 3-5 meters height. The decay of the basal portion occurs slowly and tree succumbs to the diseases in 2-3 years.

Crop stage wise IDM activities in Coconut		
Crop stage	Diseases	Step wise IDM practices
Nursery/Pre planting / Planting stage	Soil borne pathogens, wilt, nematodes	• Select good mother palm for obtaing seedlings i.e. it must be of 20 years of age, yield more than 80 nuts/ annum. • Provide proper shade, irrigation & drainage. • Rogue out diseased seedling. • Employ locally made rat traps. • Use resistant/tolerant varieties. • Sow the ecological engineering plants. • Removal and destruction of alternate host weeds. • Deep ploughing of fields during summer. • Early sowing of the crop prevents it from nematode infestation. • Liming the soil to pH 6.0-7.0, as well as reducing nitrogen levels in the soil, significantly reduces wilt.

Growth stage	Bud rot	• Adopt proper spacing and avoid over-crowding in bud rot prone gardens. • Spray copper oxy chloride 50% WP @ 1 Kg in 300-400 l of water/acre on the crown of the neighbouring palms as a prophylactic measure before the onset of monsoon.
	Leaf rot	• Follow common cultural, mechanical and biological practices. • Remove the rotten portions from the spear and the two adjacent leaves.
Mature palm	Stem bleeding	• Follow common cultural, mechanical and biological practices. • Along with 50 Kg organic manure, apply 5 Kg neem cake containing the antagonistic fungi, Trichoderma culture to the basin during September. • Provide adequate irrigation during summer and drainage during rainy season along with recommended fertilizer. • Destroy the chiselled materials by burning. • Avoid any mechanical injury to trunk. • Apply neem cake at the rate of 5 Kg/palm in the basin along with other organics.
	Bud rot	• Follow common cultural, mechanical and biological practices. • Same as in growth stage.
	Leaf rot	• Follow common cultural, mechanical and biological practices. • Same as in growth stage.

19.19 IDM in Potato

Sl.No	Name of disease	Causal organism
1	Late blight	*Phytophthora infestans*
2	Early blight	*Alternaria solani*
3	Black scurf	*Rhizoctonia solani*
4	Common scab	*Streptomyces scabies*
5	Brown rot	*Ralstonia solanacearum*
6	Wart	*Synchytrium endobioticum*
7	Black leg (Soft rot)	*Erwinia caratovora* subsp. *caratovora*
8	Viral diseases	
a	Mild mosaic/Interveinal mosaic	*Potato virus X*
b	Severe mosaic	*Potato virus Y*
c	Leaf roll	*Potato leaf roll virus*
9	Potato spindle tuber	viroid

Major diseases and their diagnostic symptoms

1. Late Blight – *Phytophthora infestans*

Diagnostic Symptoms

- Initially starts from leaf tips or margins and spread inward.
- Small faded green patches on upper surface of leaf which turn into brown spots.
- Downy growth of the pathogen on subsequent lower surface.
- Progressive defoliation and collapse of plants under favourable conditions.
- Water soaked stripes on stem which becomes necrotic.
- Purplish brown spots appear on skin of tubers.
- On cutting, the affected tubers show rusty brown necrosis spreading from surface to the centre.

2. Early Blight: *Alternaria solani*

Diagnostic Symptoms

- Brown-black necrotic spot-angular, oval shape characterized by concentric rings.
- The concentric ridges produce a target board effect, the most characteristic symptom of the disease.
- Several spot coalesce & spread all over the leaf.
- In severe attacks leaves shrivel and fall down.
- Infection and rotting of tubers has also been reported.

3. Black Scurf-*Rhizoctonia solani (Perfect stage-Thanetophorus cucumeris)*

Diagnostic Symptoms

- Black speck, black speck scab, russet scab on tubers.
- At the time of sprouting dark brown colour appear on the eyes.
- Affected xylem tissue causes to wilting of plants.
- Infected tuber contains russeting of the skin.
- Hard dry rot with browning on internal tissue.
- Spongy mass appear on the infected tuber.

4. Common Scab – *Streptomyces scabies*

Diagnostic Symptoms

- Small brownish and slightly raised spots on tubers.
- Spots enlarge, coalesce and become corky.
- Lesions typically possess a raised margin and slightly depressed center.
- Russet scab appears on tubers as superficial tan to brown corky lesions.
- Pitted scab is characterized by lesions with depressions beneath the tuber surface.
- Raised scab appears as cushion like warty lesions.

5. Brown Rot – *Ralstonia solanacearum*

Diagnostic Symptoms

- Characteristic symptoms are stunting, yellowing of the foliage, wilting and collapse of the whole plant.
- Browning of xylem tissue.
- Eye buds are black in colour.
- Bacteria ooze coming on infected tuber surface and emits a foul odour.

6. Wart – *Synchytrium endobioticum*

Diagnostic Symptoms

- Host cells at the point of infection are hypertrophied.
- White granular swellings form on the eyes of tubers.
- White tumour like outgrowths, called as warts, develop on stems and tubers.
- As the crop matures, warts become black and rot.
- Infected auxillary bud or the leaf is transformed into cock's comb like greenish.
- Yellow outgrowth.

7. Black Leg (Soft Rot) – *Erwinia caratovora subsp. caratovora*

Diagnostic Symptoms

- Disease occurs in two phases – Blackleg of shoots and soft rot of tubers.
- Black lesion appear on the base of the plant .
- Systemic and browning of infected tubers.
- Yellow appearance of the plant.
- Finally the plants wilt and die.
- Lenticels (water soaked brown rot). Rot and collapse of tubers.
- Soft, reddish or black ring appear on the infected tuber.

8. Viral diseases

a) Mild Mosaic/Interveinal Mosaic – (Potato virus X) PV X

Diagnostic Symptoms

- Often referred as latent potato mosaic.
- Light yellow mottling with slight crinkling on potato plants.
- Interveinal necrosis of top foliage.
- Stunting of diseases plants.
- Leaves may appear slightly rugose where strains of PV Y combines.

b) Severe Mosaic – Potato virus Y (PV Y)

- Also called potato leaf drop streak

Diagnostic Symptoms

- Chlorotic streaks on leaves which become necrotic.
- Necrosis of leaf veins and leaf drop streak.
- Interveinal necrosis and stem/petiole necrosis.
- Plant remain stunted in growth.
- Rugosity and twisting of the leaves occurs in combination with PV X and PV A.

c) Leaf Roll – *Potato leaf roll virus*

Diagnostic Symptoms

- Upward rolling of leaves, which have a stiff leathery texture.
- Plants stunted and have a stiff upright growth.
- Phloem necrosis of tubers in some varieties.

9. Potato Spindle Tuber – Viroid

Diagnostic Symptoms

- Plants appear erect, spindly and dwarfed.
- Leaves small, erect and leaflets dark green.
- Tubers elongated with tapering ends.
- Tuber eyes are numerous and more conspicuous.

Crop stage wise IDM activities in Potato		
Crop stage	Diseases	Step wise IDM practices
Off season/ pre-sowing	Soil borne pathogens, nematodes	• Summer deep ploughing. • Soil solarization during summer. • Field sanitation, rogueing. • Avoid water logged conditions in the field. • Follow crop rotation. • Apply manures and fertilizers as per soil test recommendations. • Start to grow ecological engineering plants. • Sow/plant 4 rows of maize, sorghum, bajra (pearl millet) around the potato crop field as a guard/barrier crop. • Raise African marigold in the nursery 15 days prior to sowing against cyst nematode. • Use raised seed beds of more than 35cm height (for better water drainage).
Sowing	Resting stage of the diseases, black heart/ scurf	• Use resistant/tolerant varieties. • Use healthy, certified and weed seed free tubers. • Tubers stored in oxygen deficient structures should not be used. • Treat tuber with M.E.M.C. 6% FS @ 0.415 g/ Kg tubers in 100 ml water for 3-5 minute or soaking potato seed tubers in streptocycline 40 to 100 ppm solution for half an hour prior to planting or with carbendazim 25%+ mancozeb 50% WS @ (1.5 + 3.0) to (1.75 + 3.5) for 10 Kg seed (tuber) or with carboxin 37.5% + thiram 37.5% DS@ (1.5 + 3.0) to (1.75 + 3.5) for 10 Kg seed (tuber).

Vegetative/ seed/ tuber stage	Bacterial wilt	• Use pathogen free tubers. • Disinfect the cutting knife using 1% sodium hypochlorite solution. • Apply lime (dolomite) in the soil as acidic or alkaline soil is not conducive to the bacterial wilt pathogen. • Two to three sprays of (streptomycin sulphate 9% + tetracyclin hydrocloride 1%) SP @ 40 to 50 ppm solution at an interval of 20 days. First spray 30 days after planting.
	Root-knot nematode	• Plant crop during the 2nd week of october in autumn and in early January to limit rootknot nematode infestation on tubers. • Grow one row of repellent plants like *Tagetes patula* and *T. erecta* (African marigold) in between 2 or 3 rows of potatoes.
	Root-knot nematode	• Apply NSKE 4% and neem cake @ 80 Kg/acre.
Tuber initiation	Early blight	• Follow common cultural, mechanical and biological practices • Chemical control: Spray chlorothalonil 75% WP @ 350-500 g 240-320 l of water/acre (second spray after 14 days interval) or copper oxychloride 50% WP @ 1 Kg in 300-400 l of water/acre or hexaconazole 2% SC @ 1.2 l in 200 l of water/acre (second spray after 21 days interval) or kitazin 48% EC @ 0.20% or 200 ml in 200 l of water or propineb 70% WP @ 300 g in 100 l of water or 0.30% as required depending upon crop stage and plant protection equipment used (second spray after 15 days interval) or zineb 75% WP @ 600- 800 g in 300-400 l of water/acre or captan 70% + hexaconazole 5% WP @ 200- 400 g in 200 l of water/acre (second spray after 21 days interval).

	Late blight	• Follow common cultural, mechanical and biological practices. • Use short-duration varieties. • Chemical control: Spray chlorothalonil 75% WP @ 350-500 g in 240-320 l of water/acre (second spray after 14 days interval) or copper oxychloride 50% WP @ 1 Kg in 300-400 l of water/acre or copper sulphate 2.62 % SC @ 400 ml in 200 l of water/acre (second spray after 3 days interval) or cyazafamid 34.5% SC @ 80 ml in 200 l water/acre (second spray after 27 days interval) or dimethomorph 50% WP@ 400 g in 300 l water/acre (second spray after 16 days interval) or hexaconazole 2% SC @ 1.2 l in 200 l water/acre (second spray after 21 days interval) or mandipropamid 23.4% SC @ 0.2 ml/ l in 200- 300 l of water/acre (second spray after 40 days interval) or propineb 70% WP @ 300 g in 100 l of water or 0.30% as required depending upon crop stage and plant protection equipment used (second spray after 15 days interval) or captan 70% + hexaconazole 5% WP @ 200- 400 g in 200 l of water/acre (second spray after 21 days interval) or cymoxanil 8% + mancozeb 64% WP @ 600-800 g in 200-300 l of water/acre (second spray after 10 days interval) or famoxadone 16.6% + cymoxanil 22.1% SC @ 200 ml in 200-300 l of water/acre (second spray after 27 days interval) or fenamidone 10% + mancozeb 50% WDG @ 500- 600 g in 200 l of water/acre (second spray after 30 days interval) or metalaxyl M 4% + mancozeb 64% WP @ 025% 1 Kg/ acre in 200-400 l water (second spray after 24 days interval) or metalaxyl 8% + mancozeb 64% WP @ 025% 1 Kg/ acre in 400 l water (second spray not less than7 weeks) or metiram 55% + pyraclostrobin 5% WG @ 600-700 g in 200 l water/ acre (second spray after 15 days interval) or azoxystrobin 23% SC@200 ml in 200 l of water/acre or treat tuber with carbendazim 25% + mancozeb 50% WS @ (1.5 + 3.0) to (1.75 + 3.5) for 10 Kg seed (tuber).
	Leaf curl	• Follow common cultural, mechanical and biological practices. • Use peppermint repellant plant for whitefly (vector). • Show attractant plant like French bean to attract predatory thrips.

	Aphid, thrip and leaf hopper (aphid's transmit potato virus Y (PVY) and potato leaf roll virus (PLRV), whitefly	• Follow common cultural, mechanical and biological practices • Use healthy seed, hot and cold weather cultivation, green manuring, irrigation, fertilizer application. • Plant early bulking and/or maturing cultivars to help seed production programme in areas having short aphid-free periods so that the seed crop may escape the population pressure of aphid vectors. • Biological control: Spray NSKE 5%. • Chemical control: • Apply thiamethoxam 25% WG @ 40 g in 200 l of water/acre or phorate 10% CG @ 4 Kg/ acre or soil drenching of thiamethoxam 25% WG @ 80 g in 200 l water/ acre for aphid control. • Spray carbofuran 3% CG @1.328 Kg/ acre for controlling leaf hopper. • Spray dimethoate 30% EC @ 264 ml in 200-400 l water/acre for controlling thrips.
	Wart	• Follow common cultural, mechanical and biological practices. • Adopt intercropping potato with maize or rotational crops such as bean and radish (reduce population of viable resting spores in soil).
	Scab	• Follow common cultural, mechanical and biological practices. • Use healthy tubers and treat the seed tubers with boric acid (3% for 30 minutes) before or after cold storage. • Maintain optimum soil moisture from tuber initiation. • Practice crop rotation with wheat, peas, oats, barley, lupin, soybean, sorghum, bajra and green manures crops. • Spray thiram 75% WS @ 25 g/ l water (second spray after 7-10 days interval).
	Black surf / Canker	• Follow common cultural, mechanical and biological practices. • Soak seed tubers in a solution of trisodium phosphate (90 g/l of water) one day before sowing. The tubers should be thoroughly rinsed and dried in shade.

Harvesting	Bacterial soft rot	• Physical damage must be avoided as it encourages post-harvest rots. • Before storage curing is effective and non-chemical control method can be done by exposing tubers for 5 days at 15 – 20 °C and 90 - 95% RH.
	Black heart	• Maintain cold storage at 4 °C or slightly higher. • Maintain proper aeration in the storage.

19.20 IDM in Tomato

Sl.No	Name of Disease	Causal organism
1	Damping off	*Pythium aphanidermatum*
2	Early blight	*Alternaria solani*
3	Fusarium wilt	*Fusarium oxysporum* f. sp. *lycopersici*
4	Bacterial wilt	*Burkholderia solanacearum*
5	Mosaic	Tomato mosaic virus (TMV)
6	Leaf curl virus	Tomato leaf curl virus (TLCV)

Major diseases and their diagnostic symptoms

1. Damping Off : *Pythium aphanidermatum*

Diagnostic Symptoms

- Disease occurs in two stages, i.e. the pre-emergence and the post-emergence phase.
- In the pre-emergence the seedlings are killed just before they reach the soil surface.
- The young radicle and the plumule are killed and there is complete rotting of the seedlings.
- The post-emergence phase is characterized by the infection of the young, juvenile tissues of the collar at the ground level.
- The infected tissues become soft and water soaked. The seedlings topple over or collapse.

2. Early Blight :*Alternaria solani*

Diagnostic Symptoms

- The disease occurring on the foliage at any stage of the growth.
- Initial symptom observed on the plants as small, black lesions mostly on the older foliage.
- Spots enlarge, and by the time they are one-fourth inch in diameter or larger, concentric rings can be seen in the center of the diseased area.
- Tissue surrounding the spots may turn yellow. If high temperature and humidity occur at this time, much of the foliage is killed.
- Lesions on the stems are similar to those on leaves, sometimes girdling the plant if they occur near the soil line.
- Transplants showing infection by the late blight fungus often die when set in the field. The fungus also infects the fruit, generally through the calyx or stem attachment.
- Lesions attain considerable size, usually involving nearly the entire fruit; concentric rings are also present on the fruit.

3. Fusarium Wilt: *Fusarium oxysporum* f sp *lycopersici*

Diagnostic Symptoms

- The first symptom of the disease is clearing of the veinlets and chlorosis of the leaves.
- The younger leaves may die in succession and the entire may wilt and die in a course of few days. Soon the petiole and the leaves droop and wilt.
- In young plants, symptom consists of clearing of veinlet and dropping of petioles. In field, yellowing of the lower leaves first and affected leaflets wilt and die.
- The symptoms continue in subsequent leaves. At later stage, browning of vascular system occurs.
- Plants become stunted and die.

4. Bacterial Wilt : *Burkholderia solanacearum*

Diagnostic Symptoms

- Characteristic symptoms of bacterial wilt are the rapid and complete wilting of normal grown up plants.
- Lower leaves may drop before wilting. Pathogen is mostly confined to vascular region; in advance cases, it may invade the cortex and pith and cause yellowbrown discolouration of tissues.
- Infected plant parts when cut and immersed in clear water, a white streak of bacterial ooze is seen coming out from cut ends.

5. Mosaic: *Tomato mosaic virus* (TMV)

Diagnostic Symptoms

- The disease is characterized by light and day green mottling on the leaves often accompanied by wilting of young leaves in sunny days when plants first become infected.
- The leaflets of affected leaves are usually distorted, puckered and smaller than normal. Sometimes the leaflets become indented resulting in "fern leaf" symptoms.
- The affected plant appears stunted, pale green and spindly.
- The virus is spread by contact with clothes, hand of working labour, touching of infected plants with healthy ones, plant debris and implements.

6. Leaf Curl: *Tomato leaf curl virus* (ToLCV)

Diagnostic Symptoms

- Leaf curl disease is characterized by severe stunting of the plants with downward rolling and crinkling of the leaves. The newly emerging leaves exhibit slight yellow colouration and later they also show curling symptoms.

- Older leaves become leathery and brittle. The nodes and internodes are significantly reduced in size.
- The infected plants look pale and produce more lateral branches giving a bushy appearance. The infected plants remain stunted.

7. Root Knot Nematode – *Meloidogyne Javanica*

Diagnostic Symptoms

- The disease is characterized by severe knotting of the roots.
- The first symptoms of the disease is stunting and poor fruiting.
- If the affected plants are pulled out and examined, the roots would be found severely knotted.
- In some cases the plants would show chlorosis but rarely do the plants die from nematode infection.

Crop stage wise IDM activities in Tomato		
Crop stage	Diseases	Step wise IDM practices
Off season/ pre-sowing	Soil nematodes, cutworm,	• Deep off-season/summer ploughing. • Green manuring with sunhemp in July-August.
Seed/nursery stage	Damping off, Soil nematodes	• Deep off season/summer ploughing. • Raised nursery beds (10 cm above ground level). • Soil solarisation for 2-3 weeks using 45 mm thick polythene sheet. • Seed treatment with *Trichoderma viride* 1 %• WP @ 9 g/kg of seed. • Mix entire nursery with Trichoderma @ 50 g/sq. m or drench the nursery with 3 g/litre copperoxychloride one day before sowing. • Use of nylon net (40 gauge) to avoid insect vectors like white fly. • Spray of copper oxychloride @ 3 g/L or Mancozeb + Metalaxyl @ 0.2%, if required repeat after 15 days. for damping off. • Raise marigold nursery 20 days before tomato nursery.
Main crop		• Transplant 45 day marigold seedlings in a pattern of one row of marigold for every 16 rows of tomato. • First and last row of field should be marigold.
	Leaf curl	• Raising nursery in protected condition (with net of sufficient mesh size to prevent the entry of vector, whitefly). • Seeds from disease free healthy plants should be selected for sowing. • In the nursery all the infected plants should be removed carefully and destroyed. Seedlings infected with the viral disease should not be used for transplanting. • Before transplanting dip the roots of seedlings for 15 minutes in imidacloprid 17.8 % SL @ 60-70 ml in 200 l of water/acre for management of leaf curl vector.

	Bacterial wilt	• Collection and destruction of disease affected plants. • Apply bleaching powder (6 g/plant), cow dung (50 g/plant) and irrigate. Don't allow irrigation water to seep from the infected area to healthy area while irrigating.
	Early and late blight	• Field sanitation. • Destruction of alternate hosts. • Provide light irrigation. • Chemical control Spray famoxadone 16.6% + cymoxanil 22.1% SC @ 0.1% or cymoxanil 8% + mancozeb 64% WP @ 0.2% or azoxystrobin 23% SC @ 0.1% or copper oxy chloride 50% WP @ 0.3% or metrium 75% WG @ 1000 g 0.2%.
Maturity stage	Fusarium wilt	• Seed treatment with *Trichoderma viride* 1% WP @ 9 g/kg seed. • Root zone application: Mix thoroughly 2.5 kg of the *T. viride* 1% WP in 150 kg of compost or farmyard manure and apply this mixture in the field after sowing/transplanting of crops. • Drench soil with carbendazim + mancozeb (0.2%).
	Alternaria fruit rot	• Spray carbendazim + mancozeb (0.2%) Fruit rot flowers get affected and droop off. Collection & destruction of such fruits is essential.
	Blossom end rot	• Spray calcium chloride (5 g/L) 2-3 times and zineb (2 g/L).
	Buck eye rot	• Staking of tomato plants. • Spray of Copper oxy chloride (0.3%).
	Nematodes	• Crop rotation with cereal crops. • Ecological engineering of tomato with marigold/mustard as intercrops reduces nematode population. • Nursery should be raised in nematode free sites or solarized beds. • Apply dazomet technical @ 12-16 g/acre (nursery).
	Mosaic	• Seeds from disease free healthy plants should be selected for sowing. • The seeds should be thoroughly rinsed and dried in shade. • In the nursery all the infected plants should be removed carefully and destroyed. • Seedlings infected with the viral disease should not be used for transplanting. • Crop rotation with crops other than tobacco,potato, chilli, capsicum, brinjal, and other solanaceous crops should be undertaken.

19.21 IDM in Brinjal

Sl.No	Disease	Causal organism
1	Damping off	*Phythium aphanidermatum*
2	Phomopsis fruit rot or blight	*Phomopsis vexans*
3	Collar rot	*Sclerotium rolfsii*
4	Bacterial wilt	*Pseudomonas solanacearum*
5	Little leaf	*Mycoplasma*

Major diseases and their diagnostic symptoms

1. Damping Off : *Pythium aphanidermatum*

This disease of brinjal seedlings in nursery beds, has been described under tomato diseases.

2. Phomopsis Fruit Rot or Blight – *Phomopsis vexans (P.S: Diaporthe vexans)*

Diagnostic Symptoms

- The plants are attacked at all stages of growth.
- On leaves, circular to irregular, clearly defined grayish brown spots having light centers appear. The diseased leaves become yellowish in colour and may drop off.
- Several black pycnidia can be seen on older spots.
- The lesions on stem are dark brown, round to oval and have grayish centers where pycnidia develop.At the base of the stem, the fungus causes characteristic constrictions leading to canker development and toppling of plants.
- On fruits, small pale sunken spots appear which on enlargement cover entire fruit surface. These spots become watery leading to soft rot phase of the disease. A large number of dot like pycnidia also develop on such spots.
- The infection of fruit through calyx leads to development of dry rot and fruits appear black and mummified.

3. Collar Rot –*Sclerotium rolfsii*

Diagnostic Symptoms

- The disease occasionally occurs in serious form.
- The lower portion of the stem is affected from the soil borne inoculum (sclerotia).
- Decortications is the main symptom.
- Exposure and necrosis of underlying tissues may lead to collapse of the plant.
- Near the ground surface on the stem may be seen the mycelia and sclerotia.
- Lack of plant vigour, accumulation of water around the stem, and mechanical injuries help in development of this disease.

4. Bacterial Wilt – *Pseudomonas solanacearum*

Diagnostic Symptoms

- Stunting, yellowing of the foliage and finally sudden collapse of the entire plant are the characteristic symptoms of the disease.
- Lower leaves may droop first before wilting occurs.
- The vascular system becomes brown.
- Bacterial ooze comes out from the affected parts.
- Plant show wilting symptoms at noontime will recover at nights, but die soon.

5. Little Leaf – Phytoplasma

Diagnostic Symptoms

- Small or little leaves.
- The petioles are so short that the leaves appear to be sticking to the stem.
- Affected plants have narrow, soft, smooth and yellow shorter leaves.
- Newly formed leaves are much shorter.
- Internodes of the stem are also shortened.
- Axillary buds get enlarged but their petioles and leaves also remain shortened giving the plant a bushy appearance.
- Mostly there is no flowering but if flowers are formed they remain green.
- Fruiting is rare, if any fruit is formed, it becomes hard, tough and fails to mature.
- Young fruit turns necrotic, get mummified and cling to the plant

Crop stage wise IDM activities in Brinjal		
Crop stage	Diseases	Step wise IDM practices
Off season/ Pre-sowing	Soil nematodes and pathogens	• Deep summer ploughing. • Addition of neem cake in soil @ 250 kg/ha (Sardana *et al.* 2004). • Soil solarization: Cover the beds with polythene sheet of 45 gauge (0.45 mm) thickness for three weeks before sowing for soil solarisation which will help in reducing the soil borne pathogens.
Seed/ nursery stage	Damping off, Root rot, Wilt	• Avoid excessive watering and poorly drained areas in field. • Use raised beds: more than 15 cm height is better for water drainage. • Use of plug tray method and sterilized potting mixture. • Nursery treatment: Mix 250 gm of *Trichoderma viride* 1.0% WP in 50 litre of water and drench the soil in 400 sq. mt. area.

		• Seedling root dip treatment: Mix 10 g of *Trichoderma viride* 1% WP in one l of water and dip the brinjal seedling root for 15 minutes. • use of nylon net (40 gauge) to avoid entry of sucking pests.
Main crop		
Vegetative stage	Root-knot nematode	• Seed treatment with *Trichoderma viride* @ 4 g/kg of seed. • Apply Carbofuran 3% CG @ 26,640 g/acre.
	Bacterial wilt	• Growing resistant varieties . • Crop rotation with non-solanaceous hosts. Since pathogen is soil borne, a rotation with inclusion of maize, soybean, wheat, rice, gingelly and green manuring has been found effective in reducing the disease in infested soil. • Green manuring with Brassica sp (biofumigation). • Soil solarization with a transparent polyethylene sheet (125 μm thick) for 8-10 weeks during MarchJune in nurseries. • Use neem cake. • Mix 1 kg of *Trichoderma viride* 1% WP with 25 kg FYM and broadcast uniformly over an acre of land and irrigate the field immediately.
Flowering stage/fruit formation	Little leaf	• Roguing out of affected plants. • Eradication of solanaceous weed hosts. • Plant tolerant varieties. • Vector (jassid/leaf hopper) control by spraying insecticides (see jassid/leafhopper).
	Phomopsis blight	• Procuring seeds from healthy fruits followed by hot water treatment of seed at 50°C for 30 minutes. • Avoid continuous cultivation of brinjal. • Rotation with non-solanaceous crops such as paddy - gingelly will helps to check the disease development. • Summer deep ploughing helps in reducing initial inoculums. • Removal and destruction of diseased crop debris. • Use resistant varieties. • Spray Mancozeb + Carbendazim @ 0.25%
	Alternaria and Cercospora leaf spot	• Spray Carbendazim +Mancozeb @0.25%, if required spray after 15 days.

19.22 IDM in Chilli

Sl. No	Disease	Pathogen
1	Damping off	*Pythium aphanidermatum*
2	Fruit Rot and Die Back	*Colletotrichum capsici*
3	Powdery mildew	*Leveillula taurica*
4	Bacterial leaf spot	*Xanthomonas campestris pv. vesicatoria*
5	Cercospora leaf spot:	*Cercospora capsici*
6	Fusarium wilt	*Fusarium oxysporum f.sp.capsici*
7	Viral diseases	
a	Mosaic	*Chilli mosaic virus*
b	Leaf curl	*Tobacco leaf curl virus*

Major diseases and their diagnostic symptoms

1. Damping Off –*Pythium aphanidermatum*

Diagnostic Symptoms

- Pre-emergence damping off: Seedlings disintegrate before they come out of soil surface. This is known as pre-emergence damping-off which results in poor field emergence / poor seed germination.
- Post-emergence damping off is characterised by development of disease after seedlings have emerged out of soil surface but before the stems are lignified.
- Lesion formation at collar region.
- Infected areas appear brown and water soaked.
- Plants shrivel and collapse as a result of softening of tissues.
- Infected stems become hard, thin (Wire stem symptoms) and infected seedlings topple.
- Disease appear in patches both in nursery and field beds.

2. Anthracnose or Fruit Rot and Die Back –*Colletotrichum capsici*

Diagnostic Symptoms

The disease occurs in two forms: the die back and the ripe -rot

Die back symptoms

- Small, circular to irregular, brownish black scattered spots appear on leaves.
- Severely infected leaves defoliate.
- Infection of growing tips leads to necrosis of branches from tip backwards.
- Necrotic tissues appear grayish white with black dot like acervuli in the center.
- Shedding of flowers due to the infection at pedicel and tips of branches.

Fruit symptoms

- Ripe fruits are more liable for attack than the green ones.

- Small, circular, yellowish to pinkish sunken spots appear on fruits.
- Spots increase along fruit length attaining elliptical shape.
- Severe infection result in the shrivelling and drying of fruits.
- Such fruits become white or greyish in colour and lose their pungency.
- On the surface of the lesions minute black dot like fruiting bodies called 'acervuli'.
- Develop in concentric rings and fruits appear straw coloured.
- The affected fruits may fall off subsequently.

3. Powdery Mildew –*Leveillula taurica*

Diagnostic Symptoms

- White powdery coating appears mostly on the lower surface.
- Sometimes the powdery coating can also be seen on the upper surface.
- Correspondingly on the upper surface yellow patches are seen.
- Severe infection results in the drying and shedding of affected leaves.
- Powdery growth can also be seen on young fruits, and branches.
- Diseased fruits do not grow further and may drop down.

4. Bacterial Leaf Spot – *Xanthomonas campestris pv. vesicatoria*

Diagnostic Symptoms

- The disease appears as small, circular to irregular water soaked areas or spots on the lower leaves.
- Spots become necrotic with brown center with chlorotic borders.
- Enlarged spots may develop straw coloured centres.
- Severely spotted leaves turn yellow and drop.
- Raised brown lesions appear on fruits.
- Narrow elongated lesions or streaks may develop on stems.

5. Cercospora Leaf Spot –*Cercospora capsici*

Diagnostic Symptoms

- Circular spots with brown margins appear on leaves.
- The spots enlarge and coalesce with others.
- The central portion of the spot becomes white and the leaves turn yellow and defoliate.
- Sometimes central portion of spot drops off.
- Spots also appear on stems and twigs as dark brown, irregular lesions with whitish centers.
- In severe cases die-back of twigs occur.

6. Fusarium Wilt –*Fusarium oxysporum* f.sp.*capsici*

Diagnostic Symptoms

- Characterised by wilting of the plant and upward and inward rolling of the leaves. The leaves turn yellow and die.
- Commonly appear localised areas of the field where a high percentage of the plants wilt and die, although scattered wilted plants may also occur.
- Disease symptoms are characterised by an initial slight yellowing of the foliage and wilting of the upper leaves that progress in a few days into a permanent wilt with the leaves still attached.

7. Viral diseases

a. **Mosaic Viruses**

Diagnostic Symptoms

- Light green and dark green patches on the leaves.
- These may be sunken or raised (puckering).
- The leaves are generally reduced in size and somewhat become filamentous like.
- Diseased plants produce less flowers and fruits

b. Leaf Curl

Diagnostic Symptoms

- Leaves curl towards midrib and become deformed.
- Stunted plant growth due to shortened internodes and leaves greatly reduced in size.
- Flower buds abscise before attaining full size and anthers do not contain pollen grains.
- The virus is generally transmitted by whitefly. So control measures of whitefly in this regard would be helpful.

Crop stage wise IDM activities in Chilli		
Crop stage	Diseases	Step wise IDM practices
Off season/ Pre-sowing	Soil borne fungus, nematodes, and resting stages of insects	• Deep summer ploughing. • Addition of neem cake in soil @ 250 kg/ha (Sardana et al. 2004) • Soil solarization: Cover the beds with polythene sheet of 45 gauge (0.45 mm) thickness for three weeks before sowing for soil solarisation which will help in reducing the soil borne pathogens. • In nematode severe area apply carbofuran 3% CG granules @ 26,640 g/acre

Seed/ nursery stage	Damping off,	• Avoid excessive watering and poorly drained areas in field. • Use raised beds: more than 15 cm height is better for water drainage. • Use of plug tray method and sterilized potting mixture. • Nursery treatment: Mix 250 gm of *Trichoderma viride* 1.0% WP in 50 litre of water and drench the soil in 400 sq. mt. area • Seedling root dip treatment: Mix 10 g of *Trichoderma viride* 1% WP in one l of water and dip the brinjal seedling root for 15 minutes. • Seed treatment with captan 75 WS @ 25- 30 g/kg seed. • Soil drenching with captan 75% WP @1000 g in 400 l of water/acre or
Vegetative stage	Fruit rot	• Production of pathogen-free planting materials. • Use healthy pathogen-free chilli seed. • Early removal of affected plants will control the spread of the diseases. • Transplants should be kept clean by controlling weeds and solanaceous volunteers in the vicinity of the transplant houses. • Stagnation of water should not be allowed in nursery beds and fields in order to avoid fungal infection. • The field should have good drainage and be free from infected plant debris. • For die back and fruit rot spray difenoconazole 25% EC @ 50 ml in 200 l of water/acre or hexaconazole 2% SC @ 1200 ml in 200 l of water/acre or propineb 70% WP @ 200 g in 200-300 l of water/acre or tebuconazole 25% WG @ 200-300 g in 200 l of water/acre or azoxystrobin 23% SC @ 200 ml in 200-300 l of water/acre or chlorothalonil @ 75% WP @ 320 g in 300 l of water/acre or kitazine 48% EC @ 80 ml in 200-300 l of water/acre

		• For anthracnose and fruit rot apply captan 70% + hexaconazole 5% WP @ 200-400 g in 200 l of water/ acre or copper sulphate 2.62% SC @ 400 ml in 200 l of water/acre or copper hydroxide 77% WP @ 500 ml in 200 l of water/acre
	Mosaic	• Select healthy seed for planting. • Crop rotation with non-hosts • Control perennial weed hosts. • Rogue out and destroy infected plants in early stages of infection. • Grow disease tolerant varieties. • Cover the seed bed with nylon net or paddy straw. • Seed treatment with imidacloprid 70% WS @ 10 g/kg of seed. • Apply fipronil 5% SC @ 320-400 ml in 200 l of water/ acre.
	Powdery mildew	• Spray fenarimol 12% EC @ 40 ml in 200-300 l of water/acre or flusilazole 40% EC @ 40-60 ml in 200 l of water/acre or sulphur 52% SC @ 800 ml in 160 l of water/acre or azoxystrobin 23% SC @ 200 ml in 200-300 l of water/acre or hexaconazole 2% SC @ 1200 ml in 200 l of water/acre or tebuconazole 25% WG @ 200-300 g in 200 l of water/acre
	Cercospora leaf spot	• Spray zineb 75% WP @ 600-800 g in 300-400 l of water/acre or copper oxy chloride 50% WP @ 1000 g in 300-400 l of water/acre
	Bacterial leaf spot	• Field sanitation is important. • seeds must be obtained from disease free plants. • Spray streptomycin sulfate 9% +• tetracycline hydrochloride 1% SP solution (streptocycline) 40-100 ppm in fields after the appearance of first true leaves. Two sprays of streptocycline, one before transplanting (nursery) and another after transplanting (main field)
Reproductive stage	Die back & fruit rot	• Same as in vegetative stage
	Bacterial blight	• Same as in vegetative stage

19.23 IDM in Cruciferous Vegetables

(Cabbage, Cauliflower, Knol-Khol, Radish, Broccoli)

Sl.No	Name of diseases	Causal organism
1	Damping Off	*Pythium aphinidermatum* (Eds.)Fitz.; *Rhizoctonia sonali* Kuhn
2	Club root of crucifers or Finger and toe disease	*Plasmodiophora brassicae* Woronin
3	Alternaria leaf spot	*Alternaria brassicae* (Berk.)Sacc; *A. brassicicola* (Schw.) Wiltshire
4	Black rot	*Xanthomonas campestris pv. campestris* (Dowson) Dye, *et al.*
5	Downy mildew	*Peronospora parasitica* (Pers.) Fr. Syno.
6	Powdery mildew	*Erysiphe cruciferarum* Opiz.ex Junnell

Major diseases and their diagnostic symptoms

1. Damping Off

Diagnostic Symptoms

- Damping off cabbage occurs in two stages, i.e. the pre-emergence and the post emergence phase.
- In the pre-emergence phase, the seedlings are killed just before they reach the soilsurface.
- The young radical and the plumule are killed and there is complete rotting of the seedlings.
- The post-emergence phase is characterized by the infection of the young, juvenile tissuesof the collar at the ground level.
- The infected tissues become soft and water soaked.
- The seedlings topple over.

2. Club Root of Crucifers or Finger and Toe Disease

Diagnostic Symptoms

- Stunting and yellowing of plants.
- Leaves become yellowish and wilt on hot days.
- Club like swelling of root and root lets.
- Club root is particularly prevalent on soils with a pH below 7, whereas it has been observed that the disease is often less serious on heavy soils and on soils containing little organic matter.

3. Alternaria Leaf Spot

- Common on cabbage, cauliflower and mustard.

Diagnostic Symptoms

- Spots are small, dark coloured.
- They enlarge, soon become circular & 1mm. in diameter. Under humid conditions groups of conidiophores will be formed in the spot.
- Spots develop concentric rings.
- Finally the spots coalesce leading to blighting of leaves.
- The fungus is seed borne and cause shriveling of seeds and poor germination
- Linear spots also appear on petioles, stems, pods & seeds.

4. Black Rot

- Serious on cabbage, cauliflower, knol-khol and raddish.

Diagnostic Symptoms

- First appear as chlorotic or yellow (angular) areas near the leaf margins.
- Yellow area extends to veins and midrib forming characteristic 'v' shaped chlorotic spots which later turn black.
- Veins and veinlets turn brown and finally black.
- Vascular blackening extend beyond affected veins to midrib, petiole and stem.
- In advanced stages, infection may reach the roots system and blackening of vascular bundles occurs.
- Bacterial ooze can also be seen on affected parts If the infection is early, the plants wilt and die If the infection is late plants succumb to soft rot and die.

5. Downy Mildew

- Severe in raddish, cabbage, cauliflower, mustard, and knol-khol.

Diagnostic Symptoms

- Small purplish brown spots on under surface of leaves.
- Small, pale yellow angular spots on upper surface of leaves, with downy growth on the under surface.
- The spots coalesce and the leaves shrivel and dries up prematurely In cabbage, these spots expose the heads to soft rot.
- Cauliflower curds look brownish at the tip.
- Stems show dark brown and depressed lesions or streaks which later develop downy growth of fungus.

6. Powdery Mildew

- Infects mostly cabbage and cauliflower.

Diagnostic Symptoms

- White powdery spots on the upper surface of leaves, stems, flower parts etc.
- Finally the mildew may cover the entire surface.
- Infected plants may show rotting and do not have normal growth.

Crop Stage-wise IDM activities in Cauliflower/Cabbage		
Crop/Crop stage	Diseases	Step wise IDM practices
Off season/ pre sowing	Cut worm, Soil nematodes	• Deep, off-season ploughing. • Green manuring with sunhemp in July-August.
Seed/nursery stage	Damping off,Root Rot, Nematodes, Black rot	• Raised nursery beds (10 cm above ground level). • Soil solarisation for 2-3 weeks using 45 mm polythene sheet. • Seed treatment with *Trichoderma harzianum / viride* @4 g/kg seed. • Use of nylon net (40 gauze) to avoid insect vectors like whitefly.
	Black rot	• Soil drenching with copper oxychloride @ 3 g/L of water.
	Downy mildew	• Foliar spray of Mancozeb + Metalaxyl @ 0.2%, if required repeat after 15 days.
Main Crop		• Wide spacing of 60 x 50 cm. • Growing of Indian mustard as trap crop after every 25 rows of cabbage. First and last row should be of mustard. • Erection of bird perches for hunting insects in the field.
Vegetative stage	Alternaria black spot	• Removal of basal and infected leaves. • Spray of Mancozeb+ Carbendaxim @ 0.2%.
	Downy mildew	• Foliar spray of Mancozeb + Metalaxyl @ 0.2%, if required repeat after 15 days.
Primoridial stage	Alternaria leaf spot	• Removal of infected leaves. • Spray of copper oxychloride @3 g/L.
	Black rot	• Copper oxychloride + Streptomycin sulphate @ 3 g +0.6 g/L. • Use of sticker with spray may be done.

19.24 IDM in Cucurbitaceous Vegetables

S. No	Name of diseases	Causal organism
1	Downy mildew	*Pseudoperonospora cubensis*
2	Powdery mildew	*Erysiphe cichoracearum,*
3	Anthracnose	*Colletotrichum orbiculare*
4	Cercospora leaf spot	*Cercospora citrullina, C. melonis, C. lagenarium*
5	Alternaria blight	*Alternaria cucumerina,*
6	Bacterial wilt	*Erwinia tracheiphila*

Major diseases and their diagnostic symptoms

1. Downy Mildew – *Pseudoperonospora cubensis*

Diagnostic Symptoms

- Symptoms resembling mosaic *viz*, pale green areas separated by dark green areas appear on upper surface of leaf.
- During wet season, corresponding lower surface is covered with faint purplish fungal growth.The entire leaf dries up quickly.
- Fruits produced may not mature and have a poor taste.

2. Powdery Mildew: *Erysiphe cichoracearum (Sphaerotheca fuligena)*

Diagnostic Symptoms

- The disease appear as superficial, powdery, grayish-white growth on upper leaf surfaces, petioles, and even main stems of infected plants.
- Affected areas turn yellow then brown and die.
- In dry seasons, powdery mildew can cause premature leaf drop and premature fruit ripening.

3. Anthracnose- *Colletotrichum orbiculare (= C. lagenarium)*

Diagnostic Symptoms

- Lesions can form on seedlings ,leaves petioles, stems and fruits of susceptible cucurbits.
- Sunken, elongated stem cankers are most prominent on muskmelon, though leaf and fruit lesions also occur.
- Large lesions girdle the stems and cause the vines to wilt.
- Stem cankers are less obvious on cucumbers, but leaf lesions are very distinct.
- Watermelon foliage affected by anthracnose appears scorched; sunken fruit lesions are easy to recognize.

4. Cercospora Leaf Spot: *C. citrullina, C. melonis, C. lagenarium*

Diagnostic Symptoms

- Initially minute water soaked spots appear on leaves.
- Spots enlarge rapidly and becomes circular to irregular with pale brown, tan or white centers and purple to almost black margins.
- Spots coalesce to form large blotches.
- The leaf may dry and die presenting the leaf a scorched appearance.
- Stems and fruits are also attacked.

5. Alternaria Blight - *Alternaria cucumerina*

Diagnostic Symptoms

- Lesions on leaves are the characteristic symptoms.
- Initially yellow brown, small but later turn into large, brown, necrotic areas with concentric zones.
- Muskmelons are more susceptible than other cucurbits to Alternaria blight. Often muskmelon vines will be almost completely defoliated by this disease.
- The pathogen also may cause fruit injury.

6. Bacterial Wilt- *Erwinia tracheiphila*

Diagnostic Symptoms

- Plant first appear dark green and then become necrotic as the wilt becomes irreversible.
- Wilt is more severe in the early season at rapid growth stage.
- In case of pumpkin and summer squash , plants may show dramatic wilt symptoms during the day when heat is more but partially recover by next morning.
- Leaves of affected plants become chlorotic and the margins become necrotic before the plant collapses and ultimately dies.

Crop Stage-wise IDM activities in Cucurbitaceous crop		
Crop/Crop stage	Diseases	Step wise IDM practices
Off season/ pre sowing	Soil borne fungus, nematodes, resting stages pathogens	• Deep ploughing of fields during summer. • Soil solarization: Cover the beds with polythene sheet of 45 gauge (0.45 mm) thickness for three weeks before sowing for soil solarization which will help in reducing the soil borne pathogens. • Apply neem cake/pongamia cake @ 100 kg/acre in soil at the time of last plouging or reducing nematodes, and soil borne pathogens. • Apply Trichoderma spp. @ 2.5 kg/acre along with FYM.
Vegetative stage	Fusarium wilt	• Use pathogen free seeds. • Remove and destroy the infected plants and plant debris. • Adopt crop rotation. • Avoid water stagnation and maintain proper drainage. • Use resistant varieties.
	Cercospora leaf spot	• Field sanitation. • Maintain good soil drainage and good aeration between vines. • Chemical control: Spray zineb 75% WP @ 600-800 g in 300-400 l of water/acre.
	Cucumber mosaic virus	• Raise 4 rows of barrier crops such as main or sorghum. • Avoid planting tomatoes next to cucurbits, spinach, or other vegetables and flowers susceptible to these diseases. • Control of aphids (*A. gossypii*) will help reduce the likelihood of cucumber mosaic. • Vector control by spraying imidacloprid 70% WG @ 14 g in 200 l of water/acre
	Powdery mildew	• Plant resistant varieties. • Increasing air movement inside the canopy. • Spray Mancozeb+ Carbendazim 50% WP @ 120 g in 240 l of water or or Thiophanate methyl 70% WP @ 572 g in 300-400 l of water/acre.

	Downy mildew	• Trellising cucumbers. Avoiding overhead irrigation or irrigating only in the late morning hours will limit the amount of time that leaves are wet. • Control alternate weed hosts (wild cucumber, golden creeper and volunteer cucumbers) in neighbouring fence rows and field edges. • Spray zineb 75% WP @ 600-800 g in 300-400 l of water/acre or cymoxanil 8% + mancozeb 64% WP @ 600 g in 200-240 l of water/acre

19.25 IDM in Turmeric

Sl.No	Name of disease	Causal organism
1	Leaf spot	*Colletotrichum capsici*
2	Leaf blotch	*Taphrina maculans*
3	Rhizome rot	*Pythium graminicolum*

1. Leaf Spot -*Colletotrichum capsici*

Diagnostic Symptoms

- Initially oblong brown spots with grey centres are found on leaves.
- The spots are about 2-3 cm in width and 4-5 cm in length.
- The grey centers become thin and gets teared.
- They are surrounded by yellow halos.
- Indefinite number of spots may be found on a single leaf and as the disease advances; spots enlarge and cover a major portion of leaf blade.
- In advanced stages of disease black dots representing fungal acervuli occur in concentric rings on spot.
- Severely effected leaves dry and wilt.

2. Leaf Blotch -*Taphrina maculans*

Diagnostic Symptoms

- This disease initially appears on lower leaves in october and november.
- The disease is characterized by the appearance of several spots of 1-2 mm in width and are mostly rectangular in shape on both the surfaces of leaves, being generally numerous on the upper surface.
- They are arranged in rows along the veins.
- The spots coalesce freely and form irregular lesions.
- They first appear as pale yellow discolorations and then become dirty yellow in colour.
- The infected leaves distort and have reddish brown appearance.

3. Rhizome Rot -*Pythium graminicolum*

Diagnostic Symptoms

- Rhizome rot symptoms show up at 90-95 days age of the crop and the leaves turn yellow in colour from tip to periphery of leaf lamina.
- Initially the margins the leaves get dried up.
- Collar region of pseudo stem becomes soft and water-soaked and plants collapse.
- The rhizomes decay as a result of the attack of the fungus.

Crop stage wise IDM activities in Turmeric		
Crop stage	Diseases	Step wise IDM practices
Pre planting/ Planting	Nematode, Soil borne pathogens and other diseases	• Deep summer ploughing during summer. • Soil solarization: Cover the beds with polythene sheet of 45 gauge (0.45 mm) thickness for three weeks before sowing for soil solarization which will help in reducing the soil borne diseases.
	Rhizome rot/ soft rot	• Use of resistant varieties to rhizome wilt/ rot. • Crop rotation with maize, cotton, soybean. • Planting of disease-free seed rhizomes. • Use raised beds of 30 cm height. • Flooding treatment for 30 days. • Soil solarisation during hottest months for 60 days. • Treat the rhizomes with hot water at 51° C for 10 minutes. • Rhizomes treatment can be done by keeping them under clear polythene sheet under direct sunlight for raising the temperature 48 °C and this temperature is retained for 30 minutes. • Use bio-fumigation using cabbage and mustard plant refuses. • Use raised beds of 15-30 cm height, 1 m width and of convenient length may be prepared giving at least 50 cm spacing between beds.
	Bacterial wilt	• Soil solarisation for 60 days during summer. • Planting of disease-free seed rhizomes. • Use crop rotation with non-host crops like ragi, paddy, maize, sorghum etc. • Avoid crop rotation with tomato, potato, chillies, brinjal and peanut, as these plants are hosts for the wilt pathogen *Ralstonia solanacearum*. • Rhizome treatment with hot water 47° C for 3 minutes. • Use bio-fumigation using cabbage and mustard plant refuses. • Avoid over irrigation, and flood irrigation in disease aff ected areas. • It is sensitive to high pH (alkaline soils).
Planting/ seedling stage*	Rhizome rot/ soft rot	• Maintain proper drainage by using 30 cm raised bed and avoiding the water stagnation. • Adopt phytosanitary measures like infected plants should be uprooted and destroyed. • Adopt crop rotation with non-host crops like ragi, paddy, maize, sorghum etc.
		• Mulching with green leaves (*Lantana camara* and *Vitex negundo*) @ 4- 4.8 t/acre at the time of planting. (It is repeated @ 5 t/acre 40 and 90 days after planting).

Vegetative & rhizome development stage:	Leaf spot	• Pluck and remove the infested leaf and uproot the infested plants and destroy them. • Use proper green mulching to reduce soil splashes. Biological control. • Use of plant extracts such as garlic extracts is effective against foliar pathogens.
	Leaf blotch	• Use proper green mulching to reduce soil splashes. • Use of plant extracts such as garlic extracts is effective against foliar pathogens.
Rhizome development stage	Soft rot/ rhizome rot	• Maintain proper drainage by using 30 cm raised bed and avoiding the water stagnation. • Adopt phytosanitary measures like infected plants should be uprooted and destroyed. • Adopt crop rotation with non-host crops like ragi, paddy, maize, sorghum etc. • Mulching with green leaves (*Lantana camara and Vitex negundo*) @ 4- 4.8 t/acre is at the time of planting. (It is repeated @ 2 t/ acre 40 and 90 days after planting).
	Taphrina leaf blotch	• Field sanitation should be practiced. • Follow crop rotation with cereal and legume crops to reduce the inoculum build up.
	Colletotrichum leaf spot	• Field sanitation should be practiced. • Follow crop rotation with cereal and legume crops to reduce the inoculum build up
	Nematodes	• Uproot and destroy the infested plants. • Treat infested rhizomes with hot water (50°C) for 10 minutes, using nematode free seed rhizomes and solarizing turmeric beds for 40 days. • Intercropping of marigold. • Deep ploughing or solarized beds of infested fi elds during summer. • Follow crop rotation with cereal crops, marigold, *Chrysanthemum, Sesbania, Crotalaria* spp., *Gaillardia*, Castor bean and *Desmodium* spp., (parasitic nematodes) • Border crops: Strips of rye grass, cover crops and mulch beds (rove beetle).
		• Application of neem (*Azaradirachta indica*) seed cake 100 Kg/acre before planting.
Reproductive /maturity	Dry rot	• Field sanitation should be practiced. • Follow crop rotation with cereal and legume crops to reduce the inoculum build up.
	Leaf spot/ leaf blight/ rhizome rot	• Same as in vegetative stage.

19.26 IDM in Zinger

Sl.No	Name of diseases	Causal organism
1	Rhizome rot/soft rot	*Pythium sp.*
2	Leaf spot	*Phyllosticta zingiberi*
3	Yellows disease	*Fusarium oxysporum* f. sp. *zingiberi*
4	Banded leaf blight	*Rhizoctonia solani*
5	Cercoseptoria leaf spot	*Cercoseptoria zingiberis*
6	Bacterial wilt	*Ralstonia solanacearum*

Major diseases and their diagnostic symptoms

1. Rhizome Rot/Soft Rot – *Pythium* sp.

Diagnostic Symptoms

- The infection starts at the collar region of the pseudostems and progresses upwards as well as downwards.
- The collar region of the affected pseudostem becomes water soaked and the rotting spreads to the rhizome resulting in soft rot.
- At a later stage root infection is also noticed.
- Foliar symptoms appear as light yellowing of the tips of lower leaves which gradually spreads to the leaf blades.
- In early stages of the disease, the middle portion of the leaves remain green while the margins become yellow.
- The yellowing spreads to all leaves of the plant from the lower region upwards and is followed by drooping, withering and drying of pseudostem.

2. Leaf Spot – *Phyllosticta zingiberi*

Diagnostic Symptoms

- Initially disease appears as small, yellowish oval to elongated spots on the leaves measuring 0.5 to 1 mm.
- The spots enlarge turn to white and papery at the centre with dark brown margin surrounded by a yellow halo.
- Spots are usually isolated but under humid conditions they coalesce with one another developing towards margin forming a big lesion.
- Black minute pycnidia develop in the white papery centre of the spots which is conspicuous in the later stages of the disease.

3. Yellows Disease- *Fusarium oxysporum f.* sp. *zingiberi*

Diagnostic Symptoms

- Yellowing of leaves starting from bottom to top.
- Drying of leaves, plants look like straw.

- Tillers do not fall to the ground.
- Shriveling/shrinking of rhizomes.

4. Banded Leaf Blight-*Rhizoctonia solani*

Diagnostic Symptoms

- Distinct irregular bands of white papery patches appear on leaves.
- Shredding of leaves occur giving a ragged appearance to plant.
- At the end, plant becomes naked with only petioles left out.

5. Cercoseptoria Leaf Spot- *Cercoseptoria zingiberis*

Diagnostic Symptoms

- Elongated yellowish brown lesions occur, running parallel to the leafveins.
- The spots are white with dark brown margins.
- Black dot like structures are seen on the white portion of the spot.

6. Bacterial Wilt-*Ralstonia solanacearum*

Diagnostic Symptoms

- No yellowing of leaves.
- Mostly drooping and downward rolling of leaves is seen.
- Neck region is not soft.
- Stem cannot be pulled out easily.
- Most of the affected tillers remain in standing position.
- Leaves turn pale green.
- Milky ooze of bacteria is very clear from cut end of tiller.

Crop stage wise IDM activities in Ginger		
Crop stage	Diseases/ Pathogen	Step wise IDM practices
Pre planting/Planting	Resting stages of diseases and nematodes	• Deep ploughing during summer. • Use of disease free planting material. • Soil solarization: Cover the beds with polythene sheet of 45 gauge (0.45 mm) thickness for three weeks before sowing for soil solarization which will help in reducing the soil borne pathogens. • Apply neem cake @ 8 qt/ acre. • Chemical control: Treat rhizomes with mancozeb+ carbendazim 50% @ 240 g/acre in 120 liter of water for 4.8-5.6 quintal rhizome for controlling yellow disease.

	Soft rot/ yellows	• Use of resistant/tolerant varieties to rhizome wilt/ rot. • Crop rotation with maize, cotton, soybean. • Plant disease free seed rhizomes. • Use raised beds. • Flooding treatment for 30 days, soil solarization during hottest months for 60 days. • Treat the rhizomes with hot water at 47° C for 30 minutes. • Use bio-fumigation using cabbage and mustard plant refuses. • Application of pine needle or neem cake powder treatments @ 0.8t/acre. • Drench affected and surrounded beds with mancozeb+ carbendazim 0.3% to reduce the spread of the yellow disease.
	Bacterial wilt	• Soil solarisation for 60 days during summer. • Planting of disease-free seed rhizomes. • Use crop rotation with non-host crops like ragi, paddy, maize, sorghum etc. • Avoid crop rotation with tomato, potato, chillies, brinjal and peanut, as these plants are hosts for the wilt pathogen *Ralstonia solanacearum*. • Rhizome treatment with hot water 47°C for 3 minutes. • Use bio-fumigation using cabbage and mustard plant refuses.
	Nematodes	• Intercropping of marigold. • Deep ploughing or solarized beds of infested fields during summer. • Grow repellant plants: Marigold, Gliricidia, Asparagus, Dahelia.
Vegetative stage	Soft rot	• Ensure proper drainage. • Adopt phytosanitary measures like infected plants should be uprooted and destroyed. • Mulching with green leaves (*Vitex negundo*)@ 4-4.8 t/acre is at the time of planting (it is repeated @ 2 t/acre 40 and 90 days after planting). Biological control: • Cow dung slurry or liquid manure may be poured on the beds after each mulching to enhance microbial activity and nutrient availability.
	Bacterial wilt	• Ensure proper drainage. • Ensure crop rotation with cereal crops.

Rhizome development stage	Leaf spot	• Pluck and remove the leaf and or uproot the infected plants and destroy it. • Use proper green mulching to reduce soil splashes. • Provide shade 30-40% to minimize the disease.
	Soft rot	• Maintain proper drainage. • Adopt phytosanitary measures like infected plants should be uprooted and destroyed. • Mulching with green leaves (*Vitex negundo*)@ 4-4.8 t/acre is at the time of planting. (It is repeated @ 2 t/acre 40 and 90 days after planting).
	Nematodes	• Uproot and destroy the infested plants. • Intercropping with marigold. • Deep ploughing or solarized beds of infested fields during summer. • Grow repellant plants: Marigold, Gliricidia, Asparagus, Dahelia. • Follow crop rotation with cereal crops, Marigold, Chrysanthemum, Sesbania, Crotalaria spp., Gaillardia, Castor Bean and Desmodium spp. (Parasitic nematodes). • Application of neem (*Azaradirachta indica*) seed cake 0.8 t/acre before planting.

19.27 IDM in Coffee

Sl.No	Name of Disease	Causal Organism
1	Rust/Oriental leaf disease	*Hemileia vastatrix*
2	Black rot or Koleroga	*Corticium salmonicolor*
3	Die back or Anthracnose	*Colletotrichum coffeanum*
4	Damping off / Collar rot	*Rhizocotonia solani*
5	Berry blotch	*Cercospora coffeicola*

Major diseases and their diagnostic symptoms

1. Coffee rust/Oriental Leaf Disease – *Hemileia vastatrix*

Diagnostic Symptoms

- The disease is restricted to leaves although sometimes it can seen on tender shoots and berries.
- The rust pustules appear as small spots, 1-2 mm in diameter.
- In early stages these spots are yellowish becoming orange in color with increase in size.
- On the upper surface, opposite the spots on the lower surface , the color is often brownish.
- In severe attack leaves may dry and wither.
- The berries remain small and fail to ripen.
- Extensive defoliation weakens the trees and results in poor yield, severe die back of twigs, and death of trees.

2. Black Rot or Koleroga - *Corticium salmonicolor*

Diagnostic Symptoms

- Dark brown or black decaying of leaves, twings and berries.
- Affected leaves get detached and hang down by means of slimy fungal strands.
- Blackening and rotting of affected leaves, young twigs and berries.
- Defoliation and berry drop occur.

3. Die back or Anthracnose – *Colletotrichum coffeanum*

Diagnostic Symptoms

- Circular to grayish spots of 2-3 mm in diameter appear on leaves.
- Small dark coloured sunken spots are farmed on berries.
- Beans become brown.
- Die back also occurs.

4. Damping off / Collar rot – *Rhizoctonia solani*

Diagnostic Symptoms

- It caused pre emergence damping off and post emergence damping off.
- In post emergence damping off collar region near soil level is infected leading the rotting of tissue and death of seedlings.

5. Berry Blotch: *Cercospora cofficola*

Diagnostic Symptoms

- Necrotic spots on the exposed surface of green berries enlarge and cover the major portion.
- Fruit skin shrivels and sticks fast.

Crop stage wise IDM activities in Coffee		
Crop stage	Diseases	Step wise IDM practices
Pre planting	Soil borne pathogens	• Deep ploughing of fields during summer to control. nematodes population, to expose popagules of soil borne pathogens. • Use virgin soil for preparation of nurseries. • Nurseries should be located far away from infested plantations. • Field sanitation, rogueing. • Destroy the alternate host plants as well as crop debris. • Crop rotation with non-cereals.
Nurseries	Damping off	• Ploughing the field before digging the pits. • Apply nutrients on the basis of soil test report and recommendation for the agro-climatic zone. • Do not re-use old nursery soil. • Avoid excess humidity in the nursery. • Disinfect soil prior to seeding. • If the disease appears, affected seedlings and those surrounding them should be destroyed.
	Brown eye spot	• Improvement of tree nutrition and shading should be sufficient to control the disease.
Young coffee plantations	Leaf rust	• Wider spacing and appropriate pruning. • Spray copper oxychloride 50% WP 1.5-2.2 kg in 300-400 l of water/acre.
	Berry disease	• Provide recommended spacing specific to varieties. • Assure proper shade. • Avoid retaining of infected berries.
	Wilt	• Promote resistant varieties. • Use disease free planting materials. • Uproot and destroy the infected trees. • Make a trench around the trees to depth of 30 cm and make sure the soil should be inside the circle.

	Stem canker	• Promote resistant varieties. • Use disease free planting materials. • Uproot and destroy the infected trees. • Make a trench around the trees to depth of 30 cm and make sure the soil should be inside the circle.
	Brown eye spot	• Improvement of tree nutrition and shading should be sufficient to control the disease.
Maturity/ Flowering	Black rot	• Removal of diseased portions. • Spray Copper oxy chloride 50% WP 1.5-2.2 Kg in 300-400 l of water/acre.
	Dieback/Anthracnose	• Follow common cultural, mechanical and biological practices.

19.28 IDM in Tea

Sl.No	Name of disease	Causal organism
1	Blister blight	*Exobasidium vexans*
2	Red rust	*Cephaleurus mycoidea*
3	Black rot	*Corticium invisum* and *C. theae*
4	Black root	*Rosellina areuata*

Major diseases and their diagnostic symptoms

1. Blister Blight – *Exobasidium vexans*

Diagnostic Symptoms

- Initially oily, yellowish, translucent spots appear on the tender leaf and turn to deep red shiny blisters.
- The circular spot gradually enlarges to 3 to 13mm diameter, bulged on the under surface of the leaf with a concave trough like depression on the upper surface.
- Leaves become curled and distorted.
- First flush of 2-3 young leaves are attacked and the young shoots and buds are killed.
- Mature leaf is not affected.
- In nursery infection, seedlings are stunted with many thin stems instead of a single stalk.
- Repeated attacks cause death of seedlings.
- Badly affected nurseries will have to be abandoned.
- Succulent leaves and green shoots of newly pruned tea are most susceptible.
- Basidiospores cause secondary infection.

2. Red Rust – *Cephaleurus mycoidea*

Diagnostic Symptoms

- Orange yellow, circular patches appear on upper surface of leaves. They are roundish in shape. Spots become brown and dry up. Reddish hairs like structure develop on the leaves. When it affects the given stem ithardens prematurely.

3. Black Rot - *Corticium invisum* and *C. theae*

Diagnostic Symptoms

- Small dark brown irregular spots appear on leaf.
- They coalesce to produce a dark brown patch which eventually covers the whole leaf and drop off.
- Before the leaf turns black the lower surface assumes a white powdery appearance.

4. Black Root –*Rosellina areuata*

Diagnostic Symptoms

- The fungus originate from the dead heaped leaves of 5 – 7.5 above the soil level.
- From there if spreads to roots region of tea bushes.
- Star like growth of mycelium can be seen when bark is removed.
- The mycelium surrounds the stem at the surface of the soil and kills the bank for the length of 7.5 – 10.0 cm.
- A swollen ring of tissue is formed round the stem above the dead patch.

Crop stage wise IDM activities in Tea		
Crop stage	Diseases	Step wise IDM practices
Pre planting / Planting stage	Soil borne pathogens	• Deep ploughing of fields during summer to control nematodes population, to expose popagules of soil borne pathogens. • Soil solarization can be done for sterilizing the nursery mixture. • Timely sowing should be done. • Field sanitation, rogueing. • Destroy the alternate host plants as well as crop debris. • Crop rotation with non-cereals. • Ploughing the field before digging the pits. • Apply nutrients on the basis of soil test report and recommendation for the agro-climatic zone.
	Nematodes	• Preparation of the nursery bed should be done by harrowing and ploughing to expose and dry the un-decomposed weeds and roots of the plants. All sorts of mulching materials should be kept away from the seed nursery to avoid nematode infestation. • Plant parasitic nematodes can be killed by uniform heating (after sieving) of the soil up to 60° – 70°C for 4-5 minutes on plain tin sheets. The soil can be used after heat treatment.
		• Removal of weed hosts from nursery beds will help in minimizing the population build-up. • Soil sampling in the estates is should be systematic following appropriate procedure to avoid errors in the assessment of eelworm. • Application of Carbofuran 3% CG@ 33.10 g/plant.

Vegetative	Red, brown and black rot disease	• Uproot the infected bushes and burnt it. • Insulation of diseases patches by making trenches of 120 cm (4 feet) deep and 45 cm (1.5 feet) width surrounding the diseased plants help in the preventing the spread of primary root disease. • Spray Copper oxy chloride 50% WP @ 0.24 Kg in 50 l of water/acre.
	Blister blight	• Use spore trap/regular field assessment. • Maintain the plucking interval. • Pruning during November/December is effective to reduce the disease incidence for new clearing. • Prohibit the entry of workers of the infested section into the healthy sections.
		• Chemical control: Bitertanol 25% WP @ 80 g in 30 l of water/acre or Hexaconazole 5% EC @ 10 g in 200 ml, 70-90 with power sprayers 175-200 with knap sack sprayer or Propiconazole 25% EC @ 50-100 g in 70-100 l of watwer/acre or Streptomycin Sulphate 9% + Tetracylin hydrocloride 1% SP @ 40 gms with 350 to 420 gms copper oxychloride (50% Wettable power) in 67 liters of water per hectare.
	Red rust	• If vigour of plant is maintained by balanced nutrients, the disease is less. • As the disease starts on the onset of rain, it is desired to spray fungicide twice during the month of July/ August at 15 days intervals. Avoid plant stress. • Avoid poorly drained sites. Promote good air circulation in the plant canopy to reduce humidity and duration of leaf wetness. • Identify and correct predisposing factors such as- poor drainage, low soil fertility, particularly potash, improper soil acidity, inadequate shade and continuous use of green crops like *Tephrosia candida*, *T. vogelli* etc. in addition to pruning of severely affected sections. • Spray Copper oxy chloride 50% WP @ 0.3% . if required repeat after 15 days.
	Black rot	• Prune or skiff the severely affected sections. Improve aeration by lopping side branches and 'matidals'. Thin out dense shade and improve drainage. • Give alkaline wash after pruning. • Shorter pruning cycle helps in minimizing infestation.

	Charcoal stump rot, Collar and branch canker Grey blight, Die back	• Remove the affected portion during rejuvenation. Avoid intensive harvesting using flat shears. • Maintain a proper balance of nitrogen and potassium fertilizers. • Avoidance of predisposing factors. • Avoid mulching and fertilizer application close to the stem collar and planting in gravelly soil. • Avoid plant stress. Grow tea bushes with adequate spacing to permit air to circulate and reduce humidity and the duration of leaf wetness. • Prohibit the entry of workers of the infested section into the healthy sections. • Spray 2-4 rounds of 5% aqueous extracts of *Amphineuron opulentum*/ *Cassia alata*/ *Polygonum sinensis* at 15 days interval.
Maturity/ Flowering	Blight, Rust, Rots, Canker	• Same as vegetative stage.

Index

P

R

S

T